Becoming Citizens

The decreasing rate of involvement in organized groups and with voting by young people is a disturbing trend that perhaps can be turned around. *Becoming Citizens: Deepening the Craft of Youth Civic Engagement* brings together civic education, experiential education, and political theory to provide a revealing multiple-perspective examination of the new alternative way of practice in the youth work field called civic youth work. This helpful resource bridges the theory of civic engagement with education, ground both in extensive data, and then discuss various youth civic engagement initiatives that battle apathy and effectively invite expanded involvement by young people.

This book is a valuable resource for secondary social studies teachers; school district curriculum coordinators; youth workers; university faculty in political theory, democratic theory, youth studies, child and youth care, recreational studies, public health, education, and social work; youth and community organizers; and program directors and managers in community-based youth services.

This book was published as a special issue of *Child and Youth Services*.

Ross VeLure Roholt is Assistant Professor at the University of Minnesota, School of Social Work and Youth Studies. He has studied and consulted on youth civic engagement and participatory youth work in the United States, Northern Ireland, Ireland, Palestine and Israel.

R. W. Hildreth is Assistant Professor at Southern Illinois University, Department of Political Science. He too has studied and consulted widely on youth civic engagement, providing technical assistance to youth programs throughout the United States and internationally.

Michael Baizerman has a long and distinguished scholarly record in the Youth Studies field. As a professor at the University of Minnesota, School of Social Work, Youth Studies, he has written widely on the topic of youth, young people and youth work and has spoken widely on work with youth and youth work professional development.

Becoming Citizens

Deepening the Craft of Youth Civic Engagement

Edited by Ross VeLure Roholt, R.W. Hildreth and
Michael Baizerman

Routledge
Taylor & Francis Group
LONDON AND NEW YORK

First published 2009 by Routledge
4 Park Square, Milton Park, Abingdon, Oxon OX14 4RN
Simultaneously published in the USA and Canada
by Routledge
605 Third Avenue, New York, NY 10017

Routledge is an imprint of the Taylor & Francis Group, an Informa business

© 2009 Edited by Ross VeLure Roholt, R.W. Hildreth and Michael Baizerman

Typeset in Times by ValueChain, India

British Library Cataloguing in Publication Data
A catalogue record for this book is available from the British Library

ISBN 13: 978-0-7890-3780-0 (hbk)
ISBN 13: 978-0-7890-3781-7 (pbk)

CONTENTS

Locating Youth Civic Engagement

A PROEM

Stepping into a group, immediately the sound reaches you even before you focus your eyes on the buzz of activity. It is loud–young people are, seemingly, all talking at once yet with each other. They sit in a poorly formed circle: some sit in chairs, others are lying on the floor, a couple sit on desks, and one or two are moving–walking or pacing– while always attentive to the group discussion even if they appear to be looking out the windows, at other groups, people walking past the door to the room. Over the noise, you hear a voice ask–softer than others but present and clear, "What can we do today that will make a difference?" The conversation shifts. Now, they are proposing next steps: those they can do now, in the last half of the time they have together this week; those they can do between this time and when they meet again next week. The adult group leader tries to remind the group of their larger goal. This is met with a confused reaction: "We're trying to figure out what we can do now!" Feverously, the suggestions are thrown to the group. Again the voice, "Can someone write these down?"

The conversation softens and a task list is created, assignments chosen, and the group separates into smaller task-oriented groups. Now laughing, then focused and working–writing, drawing, typing, looking at the internet, asking fellow group members questions about how to proceed, what they talked about last week or what someone once told them a couple weeks ago. Then the time together is over. They pack up their work, take what they will work on over the next week or so, and exuberantly walk out of the room.

Imagine you were standing against the wall inside this room. What would you notice? How would you make sense of what is going on? Now, imagine you were are no longer an observer but an actual young person in the group. Would you be the one sitting on the chair, lying on the floor, laughing with others? What do you think you would notice now? Now imagine one final role shift: What if you were an adult working with this group? What would you notice now? What has changed with each shift? There are multiple perspectives to youth civic engagement: different perspectives among practitioners–youth, youth workers, teachers, administrators–and parents as well as multiple academic frames to observe, study, and make sense of youth civic engagement. This book explores these.

HOW TO READ THIS BOOK

This text has two primary audiences: youth workers (teachers, child and youth care workers, counselors, social workers, clergy) and scholars of youth civic engagement (youth work and youth studies, sociology, anthropology, political science, cultural studies, women's studies, queer studies and the like). Because of this, every chapter may not seem equally accessible to both groups of readers; some are abstract and may be taken as theoretical and hence impractical and of little value to day-to-day practice. Others may be taken as too concrete and specific and hence of little value to scholars. We approach youth civic engagement with an orientation to what scholars call praxis–to the joining of knowing to doing in concrete, specific situations. We believe that both the theoretical and the concrete must be joined and include both types of chapters as a way to join the practice and theory together.

We do this because we believe the practitioner must know the deeper sources of her or his work and its embeddedness in a larger constellation of uses, meanings, and events. The scholar must know practice and its embeddedness in each particular here and now and across these situations towards the space of general guidelines, principles, best practices, practice-wisdom, and rules of thumb. Our hope is that the practitioner and scholar can meet within a single person, as worker and text and as scholar and text.

This goal may best be met by practitioners reading in this order: Chapters 1-4, 6, 10-11, 5, 7-9 and, for scholars, reading from start to finish. The first part (chapters 2-5) represent our study of three different youth civic engagement initiatives–Public Achievement (PA), Youth in Government (YIG), and Youth Science Center (YSC). In chapters 2, 3, and 4 we discuss these initiatives from three different perspectives–the official literature and youth and adult participants. In chapter 5 we discuss the role of program evaluation in understanding these programs. Chapter 6 summarizes chapters 2-5. The second part consists in our "readings" of these three programs and youth civic engagement in general from different academic perspectives: educational theory, political theory, theories of youth, and vocation (chapters 7, 8, and 9, respectively). Chapter 10 summarizes the theoretical chapters 7-9. We conclude by offering a new perspective on youth civic engagement which we call civic youth work.

Caveat emptor! Let the buyer beware and the reader too. Ours is not a simple, straightforward review of this literature and practice from one perspective. Instead, it opens conversation about the topic as presented in conventional scholarship and in the professional literature, offering unique and multiple points of view–those of the three civic education initiatives described here, those of young people and adults telling and describing what it is like to be a person doing civic work. This conversation is deepened by our interpretations of these descriptions from different academic perspectives. This multiplicity of perspectives is designed to enrich both the theoretical and practical conversations and serves to make more choices available to the reader–a true existential act!

THE PANIC: YOUTH ARE APATHETIC!

> The United States faces a quandary about its youth, many of whom cannot fulfill their obligations as democratic citizens. Some means must be found to overcome youthful indifference to politics; otherwise, the future of America's democratic experiment looks bleak. (Bennett, 2000, p. 9)

> Indeed, it has become a commonplace that a significant proportion of young people have no party identification, are poorly informed about and lack interest in political issues, are ignorant about political process or institutions, uninterested in the outcome of elections, and uninvolved in politics. (Frazer & Emler, 1997, p. 180)

> More young Americans can name the reigning American Idol and the city where the cartoon Simpsons live than know the political party of their state's governor. (Moore, 2003, p. 32)

These quotes can be seen as examples of a moral panic (Thomson, 1998) about young people and citizenship. The outstanding fear is the future of our democracy because of youth apathy, disinterest, and noninvolvement. This moral panic is framed by the adults who say (stereotypically) that young people nowadays are not as responsible as they were in my day (Barham, 2004; Brown, 1998); they do not care about their school or neighborhood, community or their country (Danesi, 2003; Lesko, 2001), and are much more, almost totally into their friends, themselves and their electronic toys (Buckingham, 2000; Danesi, 2003; Provenzo, 1991). They are not being prepared by parents, schools, or community leaders to be active citizens. Their heroes are from music, media, and sports, not public life (Moore, 2003). They do not look-up to neighbors working to make their street safe, clean, and keep out drug dealers. They just care about themselves and having a good time. Of course there are exceptions–the young people who volunteer at the senior high-rise building or who tutor immigrant children in English, but the narratives are always about youth in general.

This story is not new and not limited to the United States (Levi & Schmitt, 1997). We can detect panic about the state of youth going back at least to fifth century Greece. It is a narrative that has been shown by Davis (1990) in the United Kingdom to become more pointed and agitated as adults' life circumstances decline. That is, young people are a screen onto which adult concerns are projected. Economic globalization, war, and terrorism are all difficult, anxiety-producing facts for adults (Boyte, 2003; Giroux, 2003). As expected in such times, adults are more likely to find, name, promote, and respond to youth problems seeing these, at such moments, as moral panics (Cohen, 1997; Thompson, 1998). So this age-old concern about youth becomes something bigger, something that grabs our attention, and argues "something needs to be done about young people today!"

One important indicator of this concern is the amount of academic scholarship given to this sociopolitical issue (Sherrod, Flanagan, Kassimir, & Syvertsen, 2006). Indeed, most academic research documents declining rates of youth political participation. By most standard measures, fewer and fewer young people are talking about, following, or participating in politics. One of the most glaring signs of youth political disengagement is steadily declining voting rates. In 1972, around 50 percent of young people aged 18-24 voted in the presidential election; by 1996 less than thirty-three percent voted (National Association of Secretaries of State, 1999). While youth voter turn-out was up slightly in the 2000 election and more so in the 2004 election, the percentage of the youth vote in relation to the total voting population did not change. Beyond not participating in formal political activities such as voting, the great majority of young people do not even seem interested in politics of any kind. The UCLA Annual Freshman Survey has found that less than 1 in 4 respondents are inclined to follow politics and only 1 in 6 regularly discuss political issues (Sax, Astin, Korn, & Mahoney, 2003). Compounding this lack of interest, American youth are generally ignorant of the basics of the American political system (Delli Carpini & Keeter, 1996; Milner, 2002; see also Bennett, 2000). Studies documenting this ignorance reveal some distressing statistics: only 37% of high school students know the term length for a U.S. representative; worse still, only 10% can name both of their senators (Delli Carpini & Keeter, 1996; National Association of Secretaries of State, 1999). Evidence like this leads

Stephen E. Bennett (1997) to draw the conclusion that "most Americans below 30 years old hate politics" (p. 47).

While we do not doubt the research findings, we believe that Bennett's conclusion is unwarranted and actually contributes to what we are calling a moral panic. While often cast as a problem of democracy, this issue–really a cluster of issues–is often framed as a youth problem (Bennett, 1997; Mattson, 2003), an education problem (Ravitch & Viteritti, 2001), a problem about "media" (Buckingham, 2000; Milner, 2002), a social problem about "society and its values" (Putnam, 2000), and as a social problem of how individualism and consumerism have displaced a community of interests and collective action (Sehr, 1997). Missing from most diagnosis and exhortations are broad and deep analysis of this moral panic as such and a subtle and nuanced appreciation of the issues that make up elite concern about whether and how young people understand and commit themselves to the civic virtue (Colby, Ehrlich, Beaumont, & Stephens, 2003) of active political engagement.

Are Youth Really Apathetic?

We believe that before declaring youth apathetic, it is first necessary to unpack notions of involvement, participation, and engagement, as well as our understandings of citizenship. Here our point is simple and clear: there is conceptual confusion in the use of the terms involvement, participation, and engagement when contrasted with the notion of "apathy," as in young people nowadays are apathetic, do not care about their school and community, and are doing nothing to make these better. Consider any issue and three stances in relation to it as shown in Table 1.

It is easy to confuse disinterest towards a particular issue with apathy towards that issue and also, in turn, confuse disinterest with non-involvement and hence with apathy. In academic terms, phenotypic identity does not mean underlying congruence or genotypic similarity. In everyday language, what may look like apathy to one observer may not in fact be considered apathy to the person being observed. Simply put, can we fully declare youth apathetic based on the fact that few vote? Might it be disinterest in this particular election, in this choice of candidates, or in the fact that candidates are not "speaking to youth?" It may be that the empirical evidence of youth apathy is a false-negative. It is highly likely that it is not the whole story. When researchers look solely at behavior (the act of voting), they subsume intention, purpose, and meaning into behavior of voting (or not voting). Would it be more fruitful to find out

TABLE 1. Considering an Issue

Positive	Neutral	Negative
Involved		Not involved
Participating		Not participating
Engaged		Not engaged
	Apathy	

what is going on with this individual, her friends, youth in this school, community and city before judging them as apathetic?

If apathy is one form of non-involvement–the absence of interest–it is reasonable to inquire into its shapes and sources: Is someone disinterested only on this issue or on all civic issues? Is it non-involvement only on this issue or on most or all issues? Is someone's disinterest a result of not liking politics and public issues or are there other reasons? It could be that some young people have never been addressed by an issue, one that compels their interest, commitment and action, specifically, some may never have been vocationally called to an active, lived sense of being a citizen.

This volume engages these topics and goes beyond them to describe and analyze three different efforts to enhance youth civic involvement, the major understanding of youth and citizens explicit and implicit in each, and how such efforts have been–and should and could be–evaluated. Finally, we propose a new youth work orientation–civic youth work– which we discuss in detail. This is a text for practitioner and scholars both.

THE COMPLEX WHOLE AND MULTIPLE PERSPECTIVES

What indeed is the concern and does it rise to the level of genuine social or political problem? What is the complex whole? And what are its constitutive themes? Clearly there is concern by civic elites, good government groups, and a variety of other groups across the political spectrum from conservative to liberal to left radical that large numbers of young people are not actively engaged in "politics" or activities they see as political (Andolina, Jenkins, Keeter, & Zukin, 2002; Bennett, 1997; Boyte, 2003).

If the major issue is phrased in terms of limited or absent youth involvement, it is important to unpack the different perspectives, discourses, and approaches to this issue. Most perspectives share a common concern about democracy, now and in the future, and about the place and roles of young people in society and in democratic civic life, now and in the future. In the remainder of the introduction we will briefly discuss three distinct issues that help make up the complex whole of youth civic engagement. We will briefly preview what we think are three key theoretical perspectives on youth, citizenship, and vocation and then preview our contributions to this emerging field–approaching youth civic engagement from the perspective of *lived citizen* and developing an orientation towards theory and practice we call *civic youth work*.

Academic Perspectives on Youth

When we talk about youth we typically have a picture in our mind of a young person. However, beyond this very general picture, scholars have been investigating the complex ways in which youth are defined and the consequences of these definitions for youth. In the most basic sense, we are interested in what local age-sex-specific socially normative roles are available and how young people take these on and live as youth. This idea of youth as a role will be linked directly to citizen as a sociopolitical role and, in turn, to age, sex, social class, and ethnic/race-specific citizen roles.

One important contribution of the literature on youth is to define youth as a social and not a biological category (James, Jenks, & Prout, 1998). As a social category, youth embodies a set of social expectations, discourses, symbols, and other cultural representations about how body-age is to be lived, that is, how to act your age (Lesko, 2001). How old you are (Hockey & James, 1993) tells a socioculturally informed person how in general you are likely to look, act, think and feel. Of course, this is always with the proviso that, for every unique particular individual, the general may not hold at all or only in part. In lay usage this is youth culture (Austin & Willard, 1998). In scholarly terms, age as such is a social category and youth is one space within that, one often framed as a stage in the life-cycle, or life-course, in social science (James, Jenks, & Prout, 1998; Wyn & White, 1997), and literature (Heins, 2001; Neubauer, 1991).

There is youth the category and youth (young people) in general who are members of that category, as an abstract, analytical youth-population and as actual persons, 12-22 years old. Some social scientists distinguish youth from adolescent and/or teenager (Wyn & White, 1997). Most would agree that there is a time/stage of life called youth(hood) similar in conception to childhood (Jenks, 1996)–a social, political, economic (Cote & Allahar, 1994) chronological age period. Developmentalists in their science call this adolescence. A young person can be said to do youth–the social age category and to be a youth: youth is performative (Baizerman, 1998).

Academic Perspectives on Citizenship

Now we turn to a preliminary look at the concept of citizen. Like youth, citizen can be understood as a discourse (Boyte, 2004; Shafir, 1998), as a set of socio-cultural and politico-cultural representations and meanings (Vincent & Plant, 1984), and as a social role (Gorham, 1992; Shafir, 1998). Now, citizen as a sociopolitical conception is age-graded, meaning there may or may not be age-specific social expectations about what citizen is. For example, we often think that you become a full citizen at the age of 21. However, in doing so we forget that this number is somewhat arbitrary (in ancient Athens and in modern East Germany 16 year olds were given "full citizenship"). Here, we can see how youth and citizen are inextricably intertwined.

Remember that all of this so far is about how social and political institutions work and their effect on youth populations and then on individual young persons. In societies and localities where there is an explicit link between, say, age and the right to vote, the point is easy to grasp. It is harder to notice when we move away from voting to lived-citizen in everyday life in school and community: How old must you be before you can volunteer in a neighborhood clean-up event, tutor children in reading, join an anti-racism demonstration, organize a school group to study animal abuse? If these were not complex enough, add to age social class, sex, race/ethnicity, place, historical moment, individual capacity, and the cluster becomes clearer: All of these are implicated in whether and how citizen is an available sociopolitical role.

To return to the moral panic of the presumption that young people in large numbers are not actively engaged in civic issues because they do not care, do not have a sense of civic responsibility, and are too individualistic and self-indulgent, among other claims. We forget that young people, 12-22 years old, are involved in a variety of civic activities as volunteers in their school, neighborhood, and community. Great numbers are also involved in family matters as baby-sitters, wage earners, caretakers of one sort or another (without our being able to document this beyond anecdotal evidence). But they are not perceived as involved because (a) the notion of "citizen" is reserved for certain types of engagement, not others; (b) some types of citizen engagement are age-graded and hence not open to young people; and (c) adults do not perceive youth involved in certain non-age-graded activities as doing and being citizen. Thus for adults to say that youth do not care and are not involved in politics is too simple, likely wrong, and helps constitute a moral panic. This may be a false-positive panic, one that looks real but in fact is not, however real it is symbolically and in its cultural meaning.

The research literature on civic engagement investigates the general youth population's knowledge, behavior, and attitudes. It also studies the effects of interventions (programs) designed to foster engagement. Alternatively, we believe that it might be fruitful to begin with actual young people and learn what they actually do in school, neighborhood, family, and the rest, what they and others call their involvement, what served to bring them to and keep them at the work, and the like. Such research would crack some of the elements of the moral panic about youth's non-involvement as citizens. In this sense, we advance a shift in perspective from "viewing" citizenship as a role or discourse towards seeing it as a mode of doing and being-in-the-world. We hope to investigate citizenship as it is lived in everyday life. We offer the concept of vocation as a way to understand this idea more clearly.

Address and Vocational Call

We all live in a community. In what ways is this community available to us? How does it address us? How are we called upon to respond to the world? These ideas make up the venerable idea of vocation. We believe vocation can help reframe the question and concern about the low level of youth civic involvement. When read in terms of vocation, youth civic engagement can usefully be understood as a dialogical relationship of address and response or call and act.

Even though vocation has its roots in religion, we believe that one vocational self is citizen, and doing and being oneself as citizen is to be living citizen–a joining of world and self (and God) through active civic engagement. Is such an understanding helpful in practical terms? Yes, we argue, because it opens a line of practical inquiry and youth work with actual young people. Do they experience any compelling invitation to engage their school, neighborhood, or community on issues which matter to them? This is an approach typically not included in developmental, psychological, or socio-political frames. However, many will object to the religious biography, connotations and typical usage of vocational call as a frame of understanding sociopolitical phenomena and group and individual action. To them, the secular idea of address and response might be acceptable.

Martin Buber, Jewish theologian and philosopher, used the notion of address and response in a religious frame to understand the relation among person, God, and world (Friedman, 1976). Here we secularize this and introduce the notion of world-address and life-response. Each of us is available, we presume, to be addressed by persons, issues, situations, conditions, and ideas in ways that we experience as compelling and as requiring us to answer, to respond: How we respond to such an address is who we are. We define ourselves, we craft ourselves in our lived-response. Existentially we author ourselves in action, one form of which is citizen: lived-self as lived-citizen. Just as a vocational call experienced and lived is detailed in a vocational narrative, so too is our address and response–the story or narrative of who we are and why. The idea of vocation puts a young person's involvement or non-involvement in a context of compelling moral claim–does the world call you to action? A young person's response to an address, like her or his response to vocational call, is also lived in everyday life–in a group, the place of lived-citizen. The spaces of citizen are the places of the everyday; citizen is lived on the plane of the mundane, the ordinary, and the everyday.

OUR PERSPECTIVE: LIVED CITIZEN

Lived citizen is a framing of youth civic engagement that places understandings of citizenship from the perspective of education, politics, youth, and vocation. It is an attempt to get at civic engagement from inside–from the young person's embodied perspective and lived-experience. It privileges meaning, embeddedness in everyday life as context for action, and the self as praxis integrated through its acts (in contrast to a being of analytical functions or to a developing human person, for example). It is an effort to find a powerful analytic frame for understanding young people who are involved in their school and community that also opens possibilities for enhancing youth's participation by civic youth workers, teachers, counselors, and adult leaders. It is a perspective that aims to be practical.

But this is not apparent at once because it is not a common, everyday way of thinking and talking, even though it is taken to be a fine description of what it is like to be a person; it tries to get at the flow of living as lived from inside the young person. In this way, it gets at what it is like to the young person involved in a public space on a meaningful issue. But this is more than a subjective perspective, although it is that in part. It is intersubjective–person-in-relation-to-others, to issue and to a deeper, social, and individual call or address to be involved. In this way, living-citizen is existential life, one which can be read through political theory (Arendt, 1958; Dewey, 1916), social theory (Kotarba & Fontana, 1984; Turner, 1996), psychological theory (Cohn, 1997), and philosophy (Luijpen & Koren, 1969).

What is it like? As will be shown with stories below which are then analyzed in this frame, lived-citizen is experiencing oneself as having to do something on a specific issue or condition because it is the right thing to do and not to do so would go against who I am, and when I work with others on this issue, I experience myself as able to make a difference, and I feel good about this and about myself. I sometimes get involved to prevent existential guilt–my lack of courage to do what I think is right, but mostly I get involved because if I did not I would not feel good about myself.

If this is a Weberian ideal-type (Weber, 1946) lived-citizen, a model of the young citizen, taken from reality and abstracted, and if we want this to be what most young people experience and feel, then how might we bring this about? If we want more than this, for example, that young people come to be seen as true contributors to civic work, come to see themselves in this way and, quite important, continue to want to be involved as they grow older and indeed, are involved over their life-courses, civic youth work can be a viable and vital facilitator of all of this.

CIVIC YOUTH WORK

We propose civic youth work as a new member of the family of work with young people, directly and on their behalf. It is a type of generic social pedagogue (Cannan, Berry, & Lyons, 1992), and club work (Gilchrist & Jeffs, 2001), the former found in the Netherlands and elsewhere in Western Europe, the latter in the UK. In the US, civic youth work is a mixed form, joining civic education to general democratic social group work practice (Konopka, 1983).

The basic idea is to prepare workers for direct work with young people in democratic ways to bring about their experience of themselves as lived-citizen and to enhance the likelihood that they will continue to be involved as active citizens over their lifetime. And for work in schools, community, work sites, and elsewhere on behalf of the idea and belief that young people can and must be invited to contribute to their life-worlds–school, community, work site–as knowledgeable, active and moral citizens while they are young people, 12-22 years old. The last chapter of the book details the ethos and expertise of this craft orientation (Bensman & Lilienfeld, 1973) and the stages of civic youth work process.

Civic youth work has a defining ethos of youth engagement and a related pedagogy–experiential education. This means that just as citizen is lived and not simply a socio-political role, one learns how to do citizen and not simply about citizen. Civic youth workers practice experiential education in working with young people doing citizen.

CONCLUSION

This introduction opened our major subjects and some of our themes within each. The succeeding chapters include others, such as the many definitions of this youth problem, a brief history of formal and informal education in classroom and community in the US, UK, and elsewhere, and an introduction, description, data analysis and critique of three models of civic education for youth civic engagement.

REFERENCES

Andolina, M., Jenkins, K., Keeter, S., & Zukin, C. (2002). Searching for the meaning of youth civic engagement: Notes from the field. *Applied Developmental Science*, *6*(4), 189-195.

Arendt, H. (1958). *The human condition*. Chicago: University of Chicago Press.

Austin, J., & Willard, M. N. (1998). *Generations of youth: Youth cultures and history in twentieth-century America*. New York: New York University Press.

Baizerman, M. (1998). It's only "human nature": Revisiting the denaturalization of adolescence. *Child & Youth Care Forum*, *28*(6), 437-444.

Barham, N. (2004). *Disconnected: Why our kids are turning their backs on everything we thought we knew*. London: Ebury Press.

Bennett, S. (1997). Why young Americans hate politics, and what we should do about it. *PS: Political Science and Politics*, *30*(1), 47-52.

Bennett, A. (2000). *Popular music and youth culture: Music, identity and place*. New York: Palgrave.

Bensman, J., & Lilienfeld, R. (1973). *Craft and consciousness*. New York: Wiley Publishers.

Boyte, H. (2003). Civic education and the new American patriotism post 9/11. *Cambridge Journal of Education*, *33*(1), 85-100.

Boyte, H. (2004). The necessity of politics. *Journal of Public Affairs*, *7*(1), 75-85.

Brown, S. (1998). *Understanding youth and crime.* Buckingham, UK: Open University Press.

Buckingham, D. (2000). *The making of citizens: Young people, news, and politics.* New York: Routledge.

Cannan, C., Berry, L., & Lyons, K. (1992). *Social Work and Europe.* London: MacMillan.

Cohen, P. (1997). *Rethinking the youth question: Education, labour, and cultural studies.* London: MacMillan Press.

Cohn, H. (1997). *Existential thought and therapeutic practice: An introduction to existential psychotheraphy.* London: Sage Publications.

Colby, A., Ehrlich, T., Beaumont, E., & Stephens, J. (2003). *Educating citizens: Preparing America's undergraduates for lives of moral and civic responsibility.* San Francisco, CA: Jossey-Bass.

Cote, J., & Allahar, A. (1994). *Generation on hold: Coming of age in the late twentieth century.* New York: New York University Press.

Danesi, M. (2003). *My son is an alien: A cultural portrait of today's youth.* New York: Rowman & Littlefield.

Davis, J. (1990). *Youth and the condition of Britian: Images of adolescent conflict.* London: Athlone.

Delli Carpini, M. X., & Keeter, S. (1996). *What Americans know about politics and why it matters.* New Haven, CT: Yale University Press.

Dewey, J. (1916). *Democracy and education.* New York: A Free Press Paperback.

Frazer, E., & Emler, N. (1997). Participation and citizenship: A new agenda for youth politics research? In J. Bynner, L. Chisholm, & A. Furlong (Eds.), *Youth, citizenship and social change in a European context.* Aldershot, UK: Ashgate Publishing Company.

Friedman, M. (1976). *Martin Buber: The life of dialogue.* Chicago: University of Chicago Press.

Gilchrist, R., & Jeffs, T. (2001). *Settlements, social change and community action: Good neighbours.* London: Jessica Kingsley.

Giroux, H. (2003). *The abandoned generation: Democracy beyond the culture of fear.* New York: Palgrave MacMillan.

Gorham, E. (1992). *National service, citizenship, and political education.* New York: State University of New York Press.

Heins, M. (2001). *Not in front of the children: "Indecency," censorship, and the innocence of youth.* New York: Hill and Wang.

Hockey, J., & James, A. (1993). *Growing up and growing old: Ageing and dependency in the life course.* London: Sage Publications.

James, A., & James, A. (2001). Tightening the net: Children, community and control. *British Journal of Sociology, 52*(2), 211-229.

James, A., Jenks, C., & Prout, A. (1998). *Theorizing childhood.* Cambridge, U.K.: Polity Press.

Jenks, C. (1996). *Childhood.* London: Routledge.

Konopka, G., (1983). *Social group work: A helping process.* New York: Prentice Hall.

Kotarba, J., & Fontana, A. (1984). *The existential self in society.* Chicago: The University of Chicago Press.

Lesko, N. (2001). *Act your age! A cultural construction of adolescence.* New York: Routledge Falmer.

Levi, G., & Schmitt, J. (1997). *A history of young people* (Vol. 1 & 2). Cambridge, MA: The Belknap Press of Harvard University Press.

Luijpen, W., & Koren, H. (1969). *A first introduction to existential phenomenology.* Pittsburgh, PA: Duquesne University Press.

Mattson, K. (2003). *Engaging youth: Combating the apathy of young Americans toward politics.* New York: Century Foundation Press.

Milner, H. (2002). *Civic literacy: How informed citizens make democracy work.* Hanover, NH: University Press of New England.

Moore, N. (2003). What happened to civics? Today's young people are way too disengaged from the political process, according to a survey by the Alliance for Representative Democracy. *State Legislatures, 29*(10), 32-35.

National Association of Secretaries of State. (1999). New millennium survey: American youth attitudes on politics, citizenship, government & voting. Accessed-January 3, 2003. http://www.stateofthevote.org/survey/index.htm.

Neubauer, J. (1991). *The fin-de-siecle culture of adolescence.* New Haven, CT: Yale University Press.

Provenzo, E. (1991). *Video kids: Making sense of Nintendo.* Cambridge, MA: Harvard University Press.

Putnam, R. (2000). *Bowling alone.* New York: Simon and Schuster Publishing.

Ravitch, D., & Viteritti, J. (2001). *Making good citizens: Education and civil society.* New Haven, CT: Yale University Press.

Sax, L., Astin, A., Korn, W. S., & Mahoney, K. M. (2003). *The American freshman: National norms for fall, 2003.* Los Angeles: Higher Education Research Institute.

Sehr, D. (1997). *Education for public democracy.* New York: State University of New York Press.

Shafir, G. (Ed.) (1998). *The citizenship debates: A reader.* Minneapolis, MN: University of Minnesota Press.

Sherrod, L., Flanagan, C., Kassimir, R., & Syvertsen, A. (2006). *Youth activism: An international encyclopedia* (Volume 1 and 2) Westport, CT: Greenwood Press.

Thompson, K. (1998). *Moral panics.* New York: Routledge.

Turner, B. (1996). *The Blackwell companion to social theory.* Oxford, UK: Blackwell Publishers.

Vincent, A., & Plant, R. (1984). *Philosophy, politics and citizenship: The life and thought of the British idealists.* Oxford, UK: Basil Blackwell.

Wyn, J., & White, R. (1997). *Rethinking youth.* London: Sage Publications, Ltd.

Official Programmatic Descriptions

INTRODUCTION

Youth civic engagement (YCE) is a family of initiatives for young people and also a field of practice. This is a complex family with scholars and practitioners organizing the field by strategies (CCFY, 2004-2005), approaches (Gibson, 2001), and pathways (Camino & Zeldin, 2002). Within each of these are organizational structures that all agree are youth civic engagement such as service learning, youth organizing and activism, and youth in organizational decision making, and there are some that only one or two analysts describe as being in the youth civic engagement family such as youth employment, youth media, and youth development. While the range is broad, all of these provide opportunities for young people to learn about and how to do citizenship, broadly defined. Our study looked at three very different youth civic engagement strategies, approaches, and pathways: a youth program in a science museum (Youth Science Center), a simulated state government assembly (Minnesota Youth-In-Government), and a small group community action initiative (Public Achievement). For each of these initiatives, what they are often depends on who you ask.

In this and the next two chapters, we describe each of the three initiatives in our study of youth civic engagement through three perspectives. Chapter 2 is the programs' self-description, the official view as presented by program staff. In Chapter 3 the same three initiatives are then described by their young participants. In Chapter 4, Public Achievement is again described, this time by the adult leaders. Within each chapter, comparisons are made across initiatives and between official, youth, and adult perspectives. This is done to draw out the many places of agreement and disagreement about what goes on in each initiative. This allows us to highlight and clarify the differences between and among the three programs. The description of each initiative details its aims, strategies, ethos, curriculum, and activities. Aims refers to the overall purposes, strategies to the ways of accomplishing these aims, ethos to the general values of the work, curriculum to the structure of learning, and activities to what young people do in these projects. Taken together in this way, full descriptions are provided of each initiative and of the three together.

Youth civic engagement is often described through adult perspectives. Adults categorize and name what these initiatives are about in scholarly research, funding applications, and resource manuals. In this chapter, the official description of these initiatives are analyzed and compared. Officially these programs are all described as being very different from each other.

OFFICIAL DESCRIPTIONS OF THE THREE INITIATIVES

In this chapter three initiatives–Youth-in-Government (YIG), the Science Museum of Minnesota's Youth Science Center (YSC) and

Public Achievement (PA)–are described using their own literature, including strategic plans, publicity materials, grant applications, and final evaluation reports. This we call the official description because it is, with the possible exception of evaluation reports, how the initiatives want to be seen and known.

Public Achievement

> Public Work is the expenditure of visible efforts by ordinary citizens whose collective labors produce things or create processes of lasting civic value. (Farr & Boyte, 1997, p. 42)

Public Achievement's (PA) aims, strategy, curriculum, and activities are described in an official PA guide, the Green Book (Hildreth, 1998), as "young people doing and learning about public work" (p. 4). PA is not a "new youth organization" but rather a "way of life" (p. 4). The strategy is learning to do this way of life. In PA, "young people learn about politics and citizenship through the actual experience of productively engaging the public world" (p. 17). This engagement takes place within small teams, typically based in schools, community centers, or at religious institutions.

Public work is also their ethos. In particular, their values include the belief that ordinary people of all ages can contribute to solving community problems and that a citizen is a "public co-creator." They take the stance that public life begins with citizens themselves and cannot be explained adequately by references to abstract democratic institutions and principles (Hildreth, 1998). In the Green Book, PA is compared to historical social movements, such as the African-American freedom movement with its Citizenship Schools. Their goal is to create a space that encourages and supports civic action (Evans & Boyte, 1986) while embodying the spirit of joint work among youth who are engaged in democratic practice and showing this in their public work in their communities.

The PA curriculum is found in the Green Book and is on their Web site (www.publicwork.org). The curriculum is carried out in six stages, around several sets of core elements.

1. Issue definition–where young people brainstorm the many different public issues they are concerned about and want to work on;
2. Issue convention–where the specific public issues are chosen and teams are formed based on individual interest;
3. Issue research;

4. Planning a group and/or individual response;
5. Acting on the plan;
6. Evaluating what they did and how they did it.

This evaluation by youth can spark the group to move through another cycle with the same stages or it can be used to re-craft the action plan, a process almost identical to action research (McNiff & Whitehead, 2002; Whyte, 1991). There are "core elements" for participants, group projects, coaches, and project sites. For young people, examples of these include voluntary participation, work done in teams of 6-8 people, and issues grounded in participants' passions. Examples of the core elements for deciding on group projects include their legality, being non-violent, and contributing to the public good. For the coach, the adult guide who supports the team of young people, core element examples include acting as a guide and not a group leader, discussing theory and practice, guided group reflection, and helping teams to do public work. Finally for sites, where the groups meet, e.g., schools, community organizations or religious spaces, the core elements are used within the official description to define site staff responsibilities including integrating the work of the groups into the larger site, providing support for the coaches and groups, and so on. These sets of core elements create a space for youth activity.

This curriculum encourages young people to carry-out a range of activities such as public speaking, doing research on an issue, using the telephone, writing letters, and planning group action. To PA, this is public work. PA is clearly action-learning (Argyris, 1993) and experiential learning (Boud, Cohen, & Walker, 1993; Kolb, 1984). But it is decidedly not "service learning"; on this the founder, Boyte (1991; Farr & Boyte, 1997), is explicit and adamant.

Youth-in-Government: Model Assembly

Officially, the aims of Youth-in-Government (YIG) are to work to "develop personal growth" in young people and "encourage life-long, responsible citizenship" (Youth-in-Government, 1997-2003a). This holds for all YIG programs, including Model Assembly, Model UN, and the national assembly. This study looked at only the Model Assembly, which has the aim of providing "hands-on opportunity for young people to learn about their government," with primary focus on the Minnesota state level (Youth-in-Government, 1997-2003b). It takes place yearly for four days at the Minnesota State Capital in St. Paul and at hotel in Minneapolis.

YIG's strategy is described as "experiential learning for young people" using "public forums to recognize the abilities and capabilities of youth." In Model Assembly, this involves a:

> ...realistic and complex simulation of Minnesota state government, involving over 1500 young people every year, [where] participants have opportunities to serve as legislators, leadership core members, judges, justices, attorneys, lobbyists, cabinet members, and to work in the offices of the Youth Attorney General and Youth Secretary of State. Students may also choose to spend their time exploring the role that media plays in the government by taking part in the production of their own daily newspaper, nightly television news broadcast, or radio station. (Youth-in-Government, 1997-2003b)

Model Assembly (MA) has a code-of-conduct and other guidelines which emphasize that this experience is serious. At MA, young people take on governmental and public roles such as senator, representative, and justice. They wear professional attire and act professional, i.e., adult like. In the YIG Binder (the four-inch, three-ring notebook), expectations are clarified; examples include: "No food, drinks, gum, tobacco or candy is allowed in any area of the Capital building" (Youth-in-Government, 2003, p. 21) and "participants must be quiet when moving between meeting rooms and on sleeping floors out of respect to other guests" (Youth-in-Government, 2003, p. 24). YIG is the only initiative of the three that charges a program fee, which is set yearly (Youth-in-Government, 1997-2003a). In 2003, typical fees paid by young people came to about $300, with scholarship assistance available.

YIG curriculum is built around this Model Assembly (MA). Beginning months before MA, young people meet with their local delegations in their local communities (typically within a single school), to work on assignments given to them. For example, this might be to write legislative bills, legal briefs, lobbyist papers, news articles or to do similar tasks as part of their assigned role in the four-day event. All delegations meet together for a one day convention (usually in October) to be trained for their assigned roles. There they meet candidates for elected positions, such as Youth Governor, Attorney General, and Secretary of State, and vote for them. All of this preparation comes together at the January MA where they present publicly what they have been working on over the last several months.

Overall, YIG is a highly formal project with a tightly defined purpose, practices, and procedures where youth are assigned roles which they take on only for this four day event. YIG is school-like but not school in its formality, procedures, and adult control. It is not real world but is a simulation. It is playing-at being in the public sphere; it is not ongoing citizen work in school or community.

Youth Science Center

The stated aim of the Youth Science Center (YSC) is to "promote the healthy development of youth by involving them in the process of science and [by] providing them with the opportunities to contribute to others while learning" (Youth Science Center, 1996, p. 1). The strategy has four elements: YSC involves "young people in the real work of the museum"; it creates "pathways to science learning throughout the region and within the Science Museum of Minnesota"; it "actively participates with public and private organizations and institutions that share its goals of promoting healthy youth development and providing young people with opportunities to participate in shaping and strengthening their community"; and it works at being "accessible and actively engaged with diverse and disadvantaged youth, families, and communities" (Youth Science Center, 1996, pp. 9-10). Young people from diverse backgrounds participate in a wide range of museum related activities such as assisting visitors, building exhibits, and doing scientific research.

YSC staff, in partnership with community youth workers, parents and involved young people created a set of principles early on that they say are basic and "critical" to their work. It is their ethos and includes learning and engagement, equality of outcome, participation and choice, responsibility and empowerment, and partnership. For example, in the recruitment brochure (Youth Science Center, n.d.) questions shape the context, emphasizing the choices young people can make as a member of YSC. Some of the options include learning new facts and theories about science, contributing to your community, and expressing yourself. In another description, YSC highlights the value of equity in science and math by committing to recruit diverse program participants, including at least 50% girls, 50% students of color and 50% students from families with low incomes (Youth Science Center, n.d.). All of these points can be directly tied to their ethos and operating principles.

The YSC curriculum is organized around four main program areas: Explainers, Project Club, Field School, and Community Science. In their own description, the curriculum and activities merge. What is learned depends on what young people are doing and the questions they ask. YSC describes the curriculum as young people working in different spaces throughout the museum and participating in different activities such as teaching workshops to children, working in museum galleries, sharing information with visitors about current exhibition, developing educational programs for other young people in surrounding communities and inside the museum, and so on. While so engaged, they have opportunity for skill and personal development. Exactly what is given and what is learned depends on what young people ask for and demonstrate a need for. In these ways, the curriculum is emergent and co-created, between young people and adults as they go about doing a variety of museum activities.

Overall, these three civic engagement initiatives differ in their goals and methods yet are surprisingly similar in expected outcomes–as seen from the perspective of the adults, using their materials and supplementing this with participant observation. This is seen in Table 2.

COMPARING OFFICIAL DESCRIPTIONS

Comparing these initiatives based on their official descriptions, they are quite different from each other. Even the two obvious youth civic engagement programs, YIG and PA, do not appear to be similar. Each

TABLE 2. Official Description of the Three Initiatives

Descriptor	Public Achievement	Youth-in-Government	Youth Science Center
Aims	Engage young people in doing and learning "public work" and produce changes in communities, broadly defined	Develop personal growth and encourage life-long, responsible citizenship	Engage teens 11-18 in science learning
Strategy	Public work: young people learn about politics and citizenship through the actual experience of productively engaging the public world	Experiential learning for young people; recognize youth abilities and capacities	Involve young people in the real work of the museum
Ethos	Public focus Co-creative	Adult Professional	Questions Collaborative
Curriculum	Green book	Mock state government YIG Notebook (2003)	Four main programs Emergent
Activities	Public work	Acting as state government officials	Real museum work

locates itself in different programmatic theoretical and language context (Camino & Zeldin, 2002; Gibson, 2001). The third program, YSC, on the surface does not even seem to fit into the family of youth civic engagement. Why is it included?

Looking beyond the official, formal language used by each in describing itself, seeking agreement on meaning, several similarities appear at once. These are summarized in Table 3. The three initiatives describe themselves as educational and all claim experiential education (Kolb, 1984) as their pedagogy, albeit with different strategies of implementing this. Of the three, YIG is distinct in how its experiential education strategy is implemented. Its pedagogy is aligned with the method of role-playing, with young people given roles they play for a weekend. The other two provide structure and support for young people to do real world work over the longer term.

The difference clearly is in the context. PA and YSC use a real world context for learning and involve young people in work that has real and public consequence. Young people involved in YSC have created exhibitions for the museum, develop and deliver science education workshops for out-of-school time programs, while young people in PA raise money to buy books for the local library, improve local parks and playgrounds, and address issues within their schools (bullying, drug and alcohol use, etc.). YIG is a simulated experience, exposing young people to roles not yet available to them because of their age. It is future oriented while the other two are in the present. In the other two initiatives, young people's roles are shaped based on what is

TABLE 3. Comparing Meaning

	Public Achievement	Youth Science Center	Youth-in-Government
Educational Pedagogy	Experiential	Experiential	Experiential
Experience Context	Real	Real	Simulated
Program Focus	Citizenship	Science	Citizenship
Activity Focus	Choice	Choice	Designated
Program Output	Internal and External	Internal and External	Internal

needed to accomplish the work-at-hand whether it is in a museum, school, or community.

YIG and PA focus on citizenship; YSC describes itself as a having a science focus. The influence of this focus on young people's project experiences is unclear. It is reasonable to expect that young people participating in YIG and PA take part in similar experiences, except that each has a very different understanding of citizenship (Gorham, 1992). YIG focuses on formal state government institutions and process while PA argues that the YIG focus does not get at citizenship (Hildreth, 1998). To PA, citizens are "public co-creators" (Boyte, 2003). Using this definition, YSC and PA are more similar, with both emphasizing young people making public contributions in the real worlds of school, community, and museum (Hildreth, 2000; Velure Roholt & Steiner, 2005).

YSC and PA also agree on activity focus, both structured so that young people themselves have a voice in determining daily activity and over an entire program cycle. Activity in YIG is designed for young people. Youth in YIG have limited choice in determining what they will do. For the other two, daily activities are negotiated between young people and adult staff with any number of options available so long as what they do benefits their overall goal.

Finally, the three initiatives show similar patterns when comparing output, the immediate result the program is seeking to produce. For YIG, this output is internal to the program–a good simulation experience in which young people learn about how their state government works. The other two want both internal and external outputs. The engagement of young people in public work (PA) or science (YSC) is the internal output, while making a public contribution is the external output for both. Public Achievement and YSC both want to invite and support young people improving their local communities. Youth-in-Government gives its attention to creating a personally meaningful learning experience for each young person. Comparing the three using only official descriptions, PA and YIG have less in common than PA and YSC. YIG stands out because of its practice of using a simulation and not co-created, real and new activity.

Now, we see that youth civic engagement does not necessarily refer to similar strategies, styles, outputs and outcomes, i.e., to similar work. Nor is it in language. Initiatives often used the same language to describe different things–citizenship in PA is quite different from citizenship in YIG. Here similarity was found in initiatives' educational approach and program focus.

REFERENCES

Argyris, C. (1993). Knowledge for action: A guide to overcoming barriers to organizational change. San Francisco: Jossey-Bass Inc.

Boud, D., Cohen, R., & Walker, D. (Eds.). (1993). Using experience for learning. Buckingham, UK: Open University Press.

Boyte, H. (1991). Community service and civic education. *Phi Delta Kappan, 72*(10), 765-767.

Boyte, H. (2003). Civic education and the new American patriotism post 9/11. Cambridge Journal of Education, *33*(1), 85-100.

Camino, L., & Zeldin, S. (2002). From periphery to center: Pathways for youth civic engagement in the day-to-day life of communities. *Applied Developmental Science, 6*(4), 213-220.

CCFY. (2004-2005). Approaches. Retrieved November 21, 2006, from http://www. ccfy.org/civic/yce_approaches.htm

Evans, S., & Boyte, H. (1986). Free spaces: The sources of democratic change in America. New York: Harper and Row.

Farr, J., & Boyte, H. (1997). The work of citizenship and the problem of service-learning. In R. Battistoni & W. Hudson (Eds.), Experiencing citizenship: Concepts and models for service-learning in political science (pp. 35-48). Washington DC: American Association for Higher Education.

Gibson, C. (2001). From inspiration to participation: A review of perspectives on youth civic engagement. New York: Carnegie Corporation of New York.

Gorham, E. (1992). National service, citizenship, and political education. New York: State University of New York Press.

Hildreth, R. (1998). Building worlds, transforming lives, making history: A guide to public achievement. Minneapolis, MN: The Center for Democracy and Citizenship.

Hildreth, R. (2000). Theorizing citizenship and evaluating public achievement. *PS: Political Science and Politics, 33*(3), 627-634.

Kolb, D. (1984). Experiential learning: Experience as the source of learning and development. Englewood Cliffs, NJ: Prentice-Hall, Inc.

Lesko, N. (2001). Act your age! A cultural construction of adolescence. New York: Routledge Falmer.

McNiff, J., & Whitehead, J. (2002). Action research: Principles and practices. New York: Taylor and Francis Publishers.

VeLure Roholt, R., & Steiner, M. A. (2005). "Not your average workplace"–the youth science center, Science Museum of Minnesota. *Curator, 48*(2), 141-157.

Whyte, W. (1991). Participatory action research. Thousand Oaks, CA: Sage Publications, Inc.

Youth-in-Government. (1997-2003a). Programs. Retrieved January 30, 2004 from http://www.mnyig.org/programs/programs_ma.html

Youth-in-Government. (1997-2003b). Mission. Retrieved January 30, 2004, from http://www.mnyig.org/about/about_mission.html

Youth-in-Government. (2003). Program Binder. Minneapolis, MN: Youth-in *Government*.

Youth Science Center. (1996). Strategic Plan. Available from Science Museum of Minnesota, 120 West Kellogg Blvd., St. Paul, MN 55102.

Youth Programmatic Descriptions

INTRODUCTION

The official descriptions presented in the previous chapter illustrate the diversity within the family of youth civic engagement initiatives, projects, and programs. The chapter illustrated how programs using similar educational methods (e.g., experiential education) can differ substantially in other ways. Official descriptions are typically used by scholars (e.g., Camino & Zeldin, 2002; Gibson, 2001), and program developers (e.g., Hildreth, 1998), to describe, analyze, or categorize youth civic engagement programs and initiatives. In this chapter we begin to show the limitations of using only official descriptions to describe youth civic engagement work. Although most official descriptions do include quotes by young people, program staff and scholars' interpretations and voices are privileged over how young people understand and make sense of these initiatives. In this chapter we bring in their voices and explore where they might agree with, disagree to, add to, or subtract from the official descriptions of their work. By doing so, we intend to broaden how these initiatives can be conceived, developed, and understood, showing also what it is like to be a young person doing this work.

We begin by presenting data from our interviews about the everyday lives of young people. From this data we move to describing these programs through young people's perspectives. Their descriptions are then compared to the official descriptions. Finally, we use young people's descriptions to compare across all three programs. By doing so, we intend to place youth civic engagement back into the context of the everyday lives of young people, enrich how these initiatives can be described and understood, and begin to notice what programmatic orientations and practices matter most to young people.

YOUNG PEOPLE'S WORLDS

Youth civic engagement scholarship (Bennett, 1997; Frazer & Emler, 1997), evaluation (Winter, 2003), and program development typically focuses on how to change young people's current political and civic knowledge, skills, behaviors, and attitudes. Given this focus, we might believe that all we have to do is get the *buggers* to care about politics! Often missing from these discussions is how youth-hood and young people have been increasingly domesticated (Prout, 2005) and regulated (James & James, 2004). Youth civic engagement involves more than young people choosing to participate in civic and political activity; these choices always take place within a context.

In what context do the young people we interviewed say they live in? They described their lives in similar ways: structured, silenced, and supportive. In the U.S., young people living in urban settings said they have very few options in their neighborhood or school. This is not surprising, given federal, state and local budget crises, with their diminishing funds for after-school and co-curricular activities. The young people we talked to in urban settings said they were usually unable to pay the now mandatory fees for participating in after-school activities. Structured worlds to urban young people meant having "nothing to do," going to school, coming home, and then have the option to sleep, watch television, or hang out with friends. This was not by choice. The world they lived in was structured by what it lacked: opportunities to participate in diverse activities.

In contrast, those from predominately middle- and upper-income neighborhoods, attending suburban high schools, described their days as full. Their schedules are busy with school, after-school activities, jobs, and for most, enrichment programs in music, art, or other academic activities, such as Saturday speech club. These activities are important, even necessary, they say because most colleges require co-curricular involvement for admission. This is why their lives are so busy. Some easily put in 15-17 hours a day, six days a week, living their adolescence, doing adolescence.

These are two poles on two parallel continua of how one's life is given over to organized, time committed activities and schedules. At one end of the continuum are those with relatively few options who are, consequently, mostly bored. At the other end are those with many options yet relatively little choice; they and/or their parents believe, and experts tell them, that these are things they have to do to get to where they want to go, always some place in the near future. At both ends and at most points between, young people are rarely invited by adults or other young people to make a contribution to something larger than self, friends, or family. Instead, they are encouraged to "stay out of the way" and continue to add to their personal experiences to improve their chances for accomplishing their future goals. As a result, young people are removed and separated from public decision making activities.

Young people also talk about living in silenced worlds where they are not consulted on decisions, even when these directly affect them. Even when consulted, the final decision remains under adults' full control, with very little space wherein young people can negotiate. This silence typically is reinforced at home, in school, and in most other places where young people are told what to do and how, not invited into discussions or participation. As a result of this exclusion, they have little practice expressing thoughtful opinions on issues, being involved in decision making, or in engaging public issues. They are marginalized in age-segregated worlds, seen as "not yet ready," have decisions made for them, and then told that they do not yet have the capacity, interest, or commitment to be meaningfully involved in issues which affect their lives at school, in the community, and in the larger world: they are double-bound, sent simultaneous, incompatible messages. Whether this consequence is read as fortuitous or as a problem for youth civic engagement and for their development and the like is an important topic.

But this does not mean they live without some support from others, the third theme. They talked about how parents, teachers, other adults, and peers support them by encouraging them to do well in school and to take on "leadership" roles made available to them. Most often it is their friends who provide invaluable support; they listen and encourage each other. The encouragement and psychological support they receive does not enlarge their worlds or broaden their understanding of options for joint, communal social action but instead has the effect of ensuring they continue to choose youth roles and work toward youth-specific goals; the support they receive encourages them to "follow the rules" of how to be a kid around here, now, with these others.

Young people talked about how they keep their opinions to themselves in school because, if these were known, other youth would see them as weird: "It's just that since we live in a small town, it's like you've always talked to the same people. So people are sorta like, 'Why is she doing that?'" They receive peer support when they continue doing what is normal and typical. For these youth, civic engagement projects are unusual opportunities; they are challenged by friends when they join one. All of this is typical and well known about school and youth culture (Aitken, 2001; Austin, Dwyer, & Freebody, 2003; Milner, 2002). Given this, it is not surprising that when they talk about what they do in these civic projects, they highlight what makes these projects like other known and accepted teen activities such as meeting interesting people and, possibly, cute girls or boys, going on field trips to interesting places and to sponsored dances or to other special events. This is how they gain friend's support for their involvement in these projects.

To learn that young people live in formalized worlds–as we all do–and, like adults, theirs are pretty small and closed boxes, is not to learn anything new; indeed this is the substance of a huge literature on youth and schools (e.g., Austin, Dwyer, & Freebody, 2003; Lesko, 2001; Way, 1998). But the purpose of presenting this was to briefly and quickly describe and understand their everyday lives, which is a different ground than simply understanding young people as being context free, as if their choices were all that mattered for understanding the three youth civic engagement initiatives. Now we present how these civic engagement programs are described and understood by young people involved in them, asking that you keep in mind this short reminder about young people's everyday worlds.

YOUTH DESCRIPTIONS

In chapter 2, we looked at how each of the three civic education initiatives presents itself to outsiders, including the young people it hopes to recruit. Now we move to youth who were recruited, to learn what they make of their choice. Table 4 summarizes what young people say are the aims, strategies, ethos, curriculum, and activities for each of the three initiatives. We elaborate on this summary by looking more closely at how participating young people described each of the initiatives within these five categories. By the end, we intend to show how their descriptions can both support and challenge the official programmatic descriptions.

Public Achievement (PA)

In its official description, PA is an experiential education initiative to teach young people about public work. For young people, PA is a unique and special opportunity where they have the opportunity to get stuff done and use their voice. For them, PA was the place where they finally got to do something about things they cared about.

Aim

Why join PA? Most young people said because "you're actually talking about something that you kinda care about." These conversations included issues adults believe to be serious as well as issues about young people's circumstances, which to them are equally important and serious. For example, the topical issues groups discussed when deciding on what to work on included domestic abuse, street safety, and raising donations for dog training scholarships at the local kennel club. While

TABLE 4. Young People's Descriptions of the Three Initiatives

Descriptor	Public Achievement	Youth-in-Government	Youth Science Center
Aims	Hangout with friends Talk about public issues Accept invite to participate Do something in the community	Career exploration Meet new people Change image of young people Improve college applications	Earn money Hang out with friends Appease their parents Have something to do
Strategy	Doing something for the community	Student-run Having a voice and expressing it	Doing real museum work Having a voice
Ethos	Voice Responsibility Cooperative	Urgent Passion Excitement	Not your typical workplace
Curriculum	Issues Projects Co-created	Done by young people Role specific Given Mock Government	Co-created Filled with choice Science focus Museum based
Activities	Deciding on a project Working on a project Figuring out if it was successful	Debating bills. Arguing court cases. Writing articles.	Outreach Exhibit development Teaching

adults might believe the first two issues are more serious than the third issue, young people treated all as equally important to them.

Working on a dog-training project might at first not seem like an important issue. But for one group member, this was an important and personal issue, chosen because of "My dog. That's how I got my dog, because the previous owners threw her out because she couldn't do any tricks." To this youth, PA provided an opportunity to talk about her dog and figure out ways to prevent what happened to her pet from happening to other animals. This was for her a salient public and private issue. For other young people, issues such as women's role in the school, child abuse, discrimination, having young people on school committees, playground equipment for the school, and getting more textbooks for their school were important, meaningful and serious and, hence, the topic of group conversation.

Some youth joined PA because their friends and/or adults invited them.

I signed up for it last year, by accident. My teacher told me to sign up for it, I can't remember exactly how it went. But I remember I put it down and he put me in this class. He–I don't know–he told me that he likes the way I speak and how I present myself to people. He said it would be a good way to do it. So I signed up for Public Achievement.

There are many different pathways to become part of PA and, for some, simply having been invited led them to the group.

Finally, young people joined PA because they saw there an opportunity to do good work in and for their community. They wanted to "help everybody else," "help families," "make a difference in the community and school," or "make a difference in the world." As a member of PA, they had the opportunity to "do things" for their community; it is a way to do "community service." While some adults may believe youth do not get involved in community service, public work, or civic engagement because they have not been adequately prepared (Butts, 1980), young people in PA instead focus on not being allowed to take part in these activities outside of PA; this opportunity is not available elsewhere in their school or community.

Comparing their take on the project to the official description, we are invited into a rich and deeper understanding of what Public Achievements stands for and how it works. First, their description provides a working definition of public work, one that can provide clear direction to others. That is, there is no litmus test for public work, with no issue being more acceptable or important than others. The group's only concern was to be able to define the issue in both public and personal terms: It has to matter to them and to others. Second, being asked to and supported in "making a difference" on a specific issue in their school or neighborhood or beyond is what young people say is unique. PA encourages and supports them "doing something" about issues important to them in ways that can have real consequences in and for their community and for themselves and related others. "We were serious about it. We actually wanted it."

Strategy

This work is done in one or more of these four ways: educating peers and other community members, collecting donations for local charitable non-profit community agencies, completing community "service," and/or working to "change the way things are done." Many youth talked about providing education to others in school or in the larger community. "The point of our presentation is to change the middle-schoolers' minds so they can go out in the real world and already have a state of mind of open-mindedness," one said. To educate their peers and the public, they created posters for public display, wrote educational plays or skits, put on public performances, and/or created educational videos.

Other young people talked about organizing donation drives for community non-profit agencies: "That's when we'll collect that money, all the money we get from the jars, and then we'll donate that." As part of PA, they organized drives for the local food shelf, personal item drives for the local women's shelter, and organized fundraising campaigns for specific local human service organizations.

Youth also said they "made a difference" by organizing and completing community "service." One group organized a school clean-up: "We ended up cleaning up the patio and we got a lot of volunteers. We got a lot of people that just came out and helped us and people that were in detention and volunteers too." Other PA groups organized neighborhood clean-ups, tutored younger kids, or served meals at a homeless shelter.

Finally, a few groups talked about working to make structural changes in the way things were done in their school and community. For example, one group worked to get students on the many committees at school:

> They're making a lot of changes at school and we have no say in it at all. So we're like, well why can't we be on some of the committees? And so we decided . . . we'll make that as a PA group then. And so we did a lot of work, and what we did is we've made a survey to ask teachers . . . , "Well do you think our input would be significant if we were on the committee?" And . . . , "Would you guys like, if we were on the committee, would you accept our information, or do you like think we're out of place?"

Another group talked about getting legislation written and passed, although this was rare. "What we did, we did take a lot of surveys and we did, we gave our information to a couple of other groups that was going to the capital to present the information to like try to have them, you know, introducing a bill like about that." Regardless of the specific strategy chosen, all youth saw PA as a space wherein they "could do things." "PA is somewhere I can accomplish things that I want to get accomplished," said one young person. They choose specific strategies instrumentally, and all of these fit the PA ethos.

Ethos

Young people describe this PA ethos as made up of individual and joint action, social responsibility and learning how to get along and work with others, youth and adult. From their perspective, PA is a place where "we all shared our ideas," making it a unique and different place in their lives. And not school: "Because it's like when you get out of class and you can go and speak your opinion instead of being taught to and it's more interesting." For many, school is a place where one is "taught to" and PA is a place to tell one's ideas and opinions. In PA young people could say what they wanted and not be told "no way." You can talk or tell what you believe. "You actually get to tell . . . people, what you want to do and . . . how you want to do it. And they won't have to say . . . no, you can't do that or something like that, like teachers would say, or something." To youth, PA is a place where they can "express themselves."

This expression took many forms. They did not have to talk, as in a classroom; instead, this was something they could choose to do. "Sometimes before I stated an opinion, I sit back and I listen to somebody's opinion first, because I might change mine later on. Normally, I'm not the first one to throw my opinion out there." Young people came to understand this way of being as "respectful."

To young people in PA, their opinions and ideas mattered. As a result, others who typically in school did not offer ideas did so. "Like I know that [student] doesn't normally speak up and say, 'Oh yeah, I need to get this done' or 'I want to change this.' But she actually put her input in and she said, 'Yeah, I have work here so we could change, so I could do it and stuff like that.'" Young people recognized the value of peer input, wanting to hear what others had to say, and then responding: real conversation, real group.

To the young people, having everyone's input was important because it ensured that the work was more likely to get done. "We knew we were gonna' have to plan a lot because we needed to get a lot of things done. But we didn't know how to get it done so we have to kind of work together and strategize like what we were gonna do to get it done and stuff." Another young person said this also helps the group.

> Yeah, everybody's always has their own input. And most likely if they have something they want to say and want to do, it's gonna' get done just because it works better to have everybody happy and agree on everything. That just makes everybody happy and makes the group work together so much better.

Young people saw PA as inviting and supporting them as a team in deciding what to work on and how to use their ideas. This made PA a meaningful experience.

PA was also a place where they as a group were responsible to keep individual team members and themselves accountable to each other.

Young Person: I could be mean if they didn't bring in their information.
Interviewer: You could! You could be a hard nose?
Young Person: Yeah.
Interviewer: Did it work?
Young Person: Sometimes.
Interviewer: Sometimes it would work? What was the result of you being a hard nose?
Young Person: They brought in their information.

Keeping the group on track was their responsibility, albeit not always an easy thing to do, and this made the work difficult at times. As one young person said, "The group was really hard to work with especially when you got people [who] just don't want to cooperate." Youth were responsible for keeping the group focused and talking to members who were "screwing around" or "acting childish." At times this meant asking someone to leave.

In PA, young people had to work with individuals they did not know personally and even those they didn't like.

Like right off the bat it was kind of weird because I knew people. I knew all the people. And there's only guys in the group so we kind of had an idea of what each other was gonna' do and stuff like that. But after we got to like, meet each other more, we found out about each other more, and we kind of started to know and, like, we could work together. But outside of school, we probably wouldn't talk to each other, but we'd work together during PA.

Even though they did not always work in groups with their friends, most young people said being in the group was a good experience. At times not knowing the others was a benefit. "I thought that it felt good to be part of a team. Where even though I may not be friends with any of the people there . . . it was better that way because it was like I could trust them all."

Teams work, youth said, because everyone accepted the same goal. "It don't really matter if you liked them or not, but if we actually want to accomplish what this group wants to do then we have to work with people that we like or don't like." What was most important, they said, was to complete the project, and this required them to share ideas, keep other group members and themselves "accountable" and in other ways make it possible to continue to work together.

Young people's description of the PA ethos deepens and expands the official statement of philosophy and goals. For them, this work begins with their choice about an issue to work on. Their experience supports the official description of PA as believing in co-creation, and they enrich this definition by adding the difficult and necessary choices each member has to make for this ethos to become a lived-philosophy, a philosophy of practice. While some PA sites limited young people's choice to particular themes, what remained important to young people was that adults took their issue as seriously as they did. From their description, the PA's living ethos was one to be taken seriously and served to make their work important to them and to others.

Curriculum

Young people said that PA was to them about *issues* and *projects*. This issue work is done through designing, planning, and doing their own project. In PA, these projects are created in youth-directed small groups, with adults acting as consultants. For young people, the PA way begins with their deciding on an issue to work on. "First we had to like do which sections we really want to be in, like child abuse and homeless and stuff," and issues are "something that you care about," "goals that aren't necessarily focused on . . . what you want to do," or something "that you think is really important." To be an issue, it must matter to them, i.e., be meaningful.

The next step is that groups form around specific issues and each group works on a project addressing their issue. "Most PA groups have projects and we were kind of under pressure to have a project because first semester we didn't even have one." PA work is project work and this young people direct and carry-out with adult consultation. "We get to make the decisions!" one young person exclaimed. Another said,

> You were more devoted to it because you know that you were gonna come out on top. No matter what you did, you would still be right. Because it's your decision! You came up with your group, it was your idea. So no matter how far you go, you still did good.

Sometimes this meant that the groups would take a day off and relax. "I mean we've stayed on topic a lot of the times, but there's those weeks when nobody wants to do anything and we sit there and tell each other what we've been doing and why we don't want to do anything." Being able to decide when to work, what to do and how to do it was a crucial aspect of PA for young people. They had control over what they worked on and how much, and learned that they became responsible for their project. Knowing that these decisions can affect the overall success of their project and whether or not they will get something done about the issue made the work real for them. No one was going to do the work for them. Of course, they did have adult support, and for many groups this made all the difference.

Each group is given an adult "coach" who provides some guidance. "[The coach] kind of got us talking to each other, like asking us different questions about what we knew about the other kid or stuff like that." At other times, adult guidance keeps the group from accomplishing their project, some said. For example, this happened to a group working on teenage pregnancy. The school principal cancelled the speaker that the group had already arranged to talk to them, and when the group asked why the speaker did not come, one member said "I don't know. The principal wouldn't tell us." But this was a rare event, with youth saying that most of these adults did offer constructive guidance to their project work.

More than anything, young people saw that limited time was the major barrier to finishing their project. Projects were always "rushed." PA weekly meetings during the academic year lasted between forty and sixty minutes, for 28-36 weeks, giving about 20-30 hours to create, design, plan and carry-out a project. This is a crucial limitation to good and complete work, in their view. This is a major issue for young people and a criticism of the PA curriculum, as they defined it. What makes PA frustrating to them is that they are not provided with adequate resources (time) to complete their projects. Surprisingly, this does not call for a change to the curriculum. Being expected to complete a project focused their work and often made the group work better. They did not have to like each other, just complete the project. However, goal direction did have some negative consequences. Because the curriculum pushes them to complete a project, they often miss the many accomplishments and public work that takes place along the way, while doing the work. These small accomplishments (learning to work with others, etc.) are rarely discussed by the group as public work, unlike the completed project. Young people want to finish a project and they also want to be recognized for the efforts they made even when they do not finish. For them, one way to move the official description closer to the young people's description of the curriculum and its main focus on learning and doing public work is to notice and name the pubic work they do get done.

Activities

Given its group project focus, most of their activities are related to this work. Deciding on the project's purpose, working together to come up with a plan, taking action based on this plan, and then figuring out if the action was successful are what young people describe as their PA work. This is how one young person described what her group did.

> We first started out in budget cut issues. Our first issue was the library and why the library was closed from schools and why we couldn't check out books. So we wanted to get some money for that. But in the end it got so complicated, so then we went to text-books. And we got a lot of info like everybody was suing [county] because they was getting more money for schools than [other suburban schools]. So we got some help. We knew if we did try to take it to the Supreme Court we would have had some back up. But in the end it got too critical in the end. We had other activities to do, so we wasn't able to really take it that far 'cause we wrote letters to the principal asking can we send out these surveys, but we never got any info. So in the end we just decided to ask our teachers that was on our committee what they thought about text-books. And they thought that they didn't have enough textbooks to issue homework. They didn't know which students would need extra work because they didn't have enough textbooks. So like if I was a student that was slow and I wasn't able to finish up all my work, they'd have to stay after school, and the teachers had meet-ings, and they said it's more complicated, so they had to copy out of the textbooks for worksheets and reading things, which is against the law or something. And in the end we talked to them and we asked them could they give us suggestions, so they was like we could ask for some grants to get at least one set of textbooks for each of the classrooms, one set of textbooks. But in the end when we went to [Community Fund], they said it was gonna be too much money 'cause the most they usually give out is $500 and we needed like . . . I think they said $3,200 to get the textbooks in the end. So then we started volunteering over at Mark Twain, and we were talking to my second grade teacher who I help out with the reading class. So in the end we thought since we was gonna' give them

some supplies, so we was gonna' go over there and deliver chalk, paper, what else . . . crayons, pencils, all this stuff. Then we found out there was gonna' be too much, we just asked for $250, and we bought a set of classroom books, the ones that are just the same book for every student in the classroom, including the teacher, and it was called "Time for All of Our Friends" because they was doing a project on frogs, so we thought they would be the best book to get for the whole class.

This is PA to engaged young people. More explicitly, young people come up with a project idea and then gather information on the topic and tell others what they learned. To do this, most used the internet, talked with someone, or conducted surveys. Research was ongoing, leading to the ongoing crafting and re-crafting of project focus, plan, and action.

Young people said they learned to be inquisitive and flexible in how they worked and had to be courageous because the project often required the unfamiliar and the difficult such as contacting community members and asking for information, writing grants, asking adults for assistance, writing letters to school, city and state leaders, creating and analyzing surveys, and so on. Their group provided them necessary support for these individual efforts.

Most of what young people talked about is missing from adult descriptions of the project. To young people, doing what adults might call small tasks and, therefore, overlooked tasks, was a big deal. It took their courage, they said, to do what adults might expect to be run-of-the-mill tasks such as calling adults on the telephone to get information for their project. Because these tasks were real, they had real consequences for the group project. Thus, young people took them seriously and, when they succeeded, it was because they had worked hard, they said. Young people engaged in Youth-in-Government talked about similar outcomes, even when their overall experience was a simulation.

Youth-in-Government (YIG)

I see it as an opportunity to learn and an opportunity to have opinions and be myself and an opportunity to really learn about government and really gain useful knowledge. (YIG Participant, 2003)

What makes Youth-in-Government important to me? Well, at first I joined it because I thought it would look good on a college entrance. But then it kind of changed to being a real good learning experience. It makes it important to me because I want to be a lawyer and a politician and in government when I grow up. (YIG Participant, 2003)

Seen in these quotes, young people participate in YIG to achieve personal, educational, and career goals, to meet new people, to learn and, although not mentioned here, to prove that young people can do real and meaningful work, thereby challenging the idea that youth are lazy, "slackers," and immature and irresponsible–not yet ready for citizen work.

Aim

Many young people said that they joined YIG because they could use it to achieve personal goals such as getting into college, gaining career experience, or to try out what is was like to take on certain roles. Most participated in YIG because "I'm really looking forward into my future." For participants, YIG was a way to figure out what they wanted to do–their vocational calling. As one participant said, "[I attend YIG] to prepare me for if I choose a career in the legal field and, if I don't like it, I don't want to make a career in it because I don't want to spend all that money for law school and find out I don't like it." Young people also took this opportunity to try out being a certain type of person, that is, to live their calling. "I don't want to be known as someone who's really dull and boring," one youth said. This included becoming "more informed" and being able to "form opinions." To all young people, YIG is an opportunity that will be helpful later.

Another reason they gave for joining YIG is to meet new people. With more than 1500 youth coming together for one weekend, young people have the opportunity to meet others from all over Minnesota. To them, this was exciting and a reason for joining. "Hanging out with people who you have something in common with even if you don't know their names, you definitely have something in common with them. So that's fun because then you're just with 1,500 people."

Finally, young people said YIG was a way to show adults that youth were competent, responsible and capable. In YIG, they want and can demonstrate their abilities, in part to challenge adult stereotypes about youth. This is something they want to do so that adults can see that "I'm not a regular teenager stereotype where we just sit around, are lazy, and do our work last minute. I'm doing something because I want to, because I guess it's important to me," as one young person said. Changing adult images of youth is a political and personal goal. "You explain what you've done and it really opens them up to think teens, well, this kid anyway isn't a slacker."

Most participated in the program because they believed the program provided future benefits such as choosing a good career, having long-term friendships, and setting themselves apart from a typical young person. Here, their aim and the official goal are quite different. For them, it had very little to do with life-long citizenship, developing a public attitude, and contributing to public good. Instead, they defined and understood the program in almost exclusively personal ways.

Strategy

From young people's perspective, YIG's strategy is to involve young people in mock state government. This is one young person's description.

> In school I listen to a bunch of people giving me lectures on science and math and a bunch of boring stuff that frankly I don't really care about. I almost fall asleep in all my classes. In this it's something like . . . they don't give you a lecture on this is what government's like, it's not like going to a giant civics class. It's like being in the government; it felt really real and it was a lot more fun. I learned a lot more about the government and how it really works behind the scenes. You see government on TV and you think okay, that job looks easy. They get up. They make a few speeches. They get told what to do, but they really don't. They have to figure out on their own how they're gonna' say all that stuff.

For a weekend, they are the government. As such, they have work to do, individual work that is publicly evaluated by other members. "It's a real government but we're youth. Just younger people running a real government." In these roles, they "wrote the articles" for the newspapers, "were on TV," "handled Supreme Court cases," "debated bills," "took on leadership roles" and "wrote opinions" for the bills. All of this work matters and is taken seriously by them largely because it is evaluated by other youth. This public evaluation gives "a new perspective on [their] work," because these peer evaluations matter, which makes their work meaningful and one's efforts consequential. To them, this evaluation has real consequences. And because it is real to them, participating in YIG is for them meaningful; they did work that meant something to them and to the other young people and to adult staff.

To youth, YIG is different than school, home, or their neighborhood. Here they are not told by adults what to do, or by "an authority that you consider your superior playing devil's advocate or saying that you're wrong. But you're on a level playing field with everyone else." Adults at the Model Assembly don't interfere.

> We have adults around to make sure we're doing . . . it's not like school where you gotta do this, you gotta do it now. It's like, okay, are you doing what you're supposed to? Good. We'll leave you now. You can go on. Do whatever. It's all student-run. There's like one adult in a room of three hundred kids. They don't interfere.

This encourages them to "express what they think"; they are in roles in which "your voice counts." Their voice counts because they are the ones running the simulated government these four days.

This work was different from most school assignments and thus is another part of YIG strategy. School work is about "learning to keep that all up there in my brain," while YIG work was more about using what you know to get quality work done. When talking about YIG work, they mentioned "teaching others," making a case that "we could explain in logical terms and not in law language," and "doing speeches." To the young people, this work was YIG's strategy put into action.

This work had immediate consequences during the four-day Mock Assembly. As an appellate lawyer for the weekend explained, what mattered was "how much work we did. Whether or not we really tried to look up the information or whether we were just slacking off and did our brief last minute. It depends on how much you study the case." They knew that not every law case is won, every bill passed, or every news article published. Only those judged by others as "best" received this honor. If young people choose to "slack off" it quickly became visible: "You would notice that, because some people don't know their case." For those who worked hard, participating in YIG was an accomplishment because, "It made me feel really good knowing that I tried my best; and even though I didn't win, I knew I can't win them all, but I had tried."

The strategy officially described as a simulated government experience is quite close to how young people described it, although for them it was more action-learning than experiential learning. This means that the locus of learning was in action, with young people coming to make sense of these experiences in personal but not necessarily political ways. The strategy young people described lack the necessary guided individual and group reflection to make it true experiential education (Joplin, 1995).

Ethos

Young people describe Model Assembly as filled with urgency, passion, and excitement: The four days sizzle! With only four days, each minute counted. "You only have four days and it seems like you just gotta party hardy and have your fun and meet all the people you can." Part of the urgency of the four days was trying to meet as many new people as possible. "It was fun talking and meeting new people. I talked to the people around me, got to know them. And that's the cool thing about Youth-in-Government, people are really open to meeting new people and finding out stuff about them." Adding to the urgency is the work. "We had our brief written; it had to be done by November 25, I think, and we got it done right the day before that. So we were a little late, but we had been working on it for about a month."

At Model Assembly this urgency is reinforced because now young people have only limited time to present their work. They talked about staying up late re-writing legal briefs based on how their case went earlier that day, pushing to get every bill presented and debated, and struggling to make sure some of the bills' language was changed in committee. "You never understand until you actually experience it, but your brain is going 120 mph."

YIG is a passionate time. They are around like-minded young people who, like them, are passionate about political issues and willing to talk about controversial political topics. "It makes it so much greater because you're with all these people that are just like you who have passion about things and care about the government and let their voice be heard" is how one young person talked about it. These are unique and atypical conversations, they say.

YIG is a youth world, a youth space, filled with so many young people from so many different cities; it has an atmosphere of excitement. "Going to Youth-in-Government are all these people who are really friendly and we're all there for like the same purpose; we want to get to know more about our government and meet new people and learn new stuff. It's like this stuff in the air, this aroma in the air, of excitement. Everywhere youth go they can meet new people and learn: knowledge and friendship result, an ideal youth happening!"

Obviously this differs from the ethos as officially described. Young people emphasize the overall goal and the work to achieve this. To them, being given required codes-of-conduct prior to the Model Assembly did not match the overall YIG ethos. They believed that this was an event during which they did not have to act like young people but instead had opportunity to act like government officials and to be, most said, who they really are. The official YIG description is built on an image of young person that these actual youth challenge and transcend during the Model Assembly.

Curriculum

To young people, YIG's curriculum is role specific, prescribed, and given, not open to co-creation and negotiation. This includes much of the overall structure, the different roles available to young people and their corresponding activities, the different spaces that are used for Model Assembly and how these can be used, and the relationships between different participants. All of these are defined, structured, and with clear boundaries set by adults. Young people know a great deal about what they will have to do before and during the four days of Model Assembly, yet within this well-defined program structure, they talk about where they have choices. They see that the role they are given can be carried out in a number of different ways. They choose to be appropriate senators, legislatures, lawyers, and judges; this they name as being responsible.

Young people describe the YIG curriculum the same as adults–a simulation of state government–with them playing roles such as senator, representative, news reporter, judge, and so on. All of those interviewed could describe this variety of roles.

> You have your legislative branches. You have your executive branch, which is like our Governor and . . . I think we have a Secretary of State, we have a Chief Judge, and we have an Attorney General. We have all those executive branches. And we have the legislative people, like the Chair. Then we have legislators. Then you have the courtrooms, we have the Supreme Court, and the Court of Appeals. It's just like a whole mini-government basically for the state of Minnesota.

In this "mock government," as many young people called it, there are clear YIG guidelines and these are the focus of preliminary meetings. "We just talked about the rules a lot in the meetings before [the Model Assembly]. We went over the code-of-conduct probably ten times." To them this focus on rules and clear expectations was at times both helpful and "getting in the way." "We had guidelines. We knew what we were supposed to be doing. And we all had the same sheet of paper that said the same thing. So that helped us because we could be like, you're the speaker, you're supposed to do this." Youth found it helpful that everyone understood in the same way the system they all had to work within. Did this emphasis make YIG too school-like?

No, but youth said that this focus on rules and the code-of-conduct was at times taken too far and this caused annoyance and frustration with the initiative and the adults supervising them. "Like the procedures thing I didn't like at all. It just bothers me, because I think that it isolates a lot of people. I think it intimidates people to the point where they won't stand up and say something, when you stress procedures so much." Having clear guidelines served to keep everyone on the same programmatic page but it also had negative consequences; those who did not fully understand the guidelines often were uncomfortable participating.

These guidelines and rules were elements of the simulated roles, practices, sites, and settings. Young people valued being in "actual courtrooms" and "actual chambers," because these made the simulation more real; they were "doing government." Being in the senate chambers, meeting rooms, courtrooms and other official sites of state government also added seriousness to the experience as did dressing professionally.

> I think when you put on–this sounds superficial–but when you put on the dress clothes and you're walking through with your notebook and your pad of paper and you're just like walking through a courtroom that big, with big ceilings, there's so many people and especially when you're in the front of the room, you just feel like you stand above the rest of them.

There were also times when they had options, such as debating or voting on bills. "It was fun because you can hear both sides and everything, and the thing about it is I could step down if I wanted and vote or debate on the bills if I wanted." Others talked about choices in how they played their YIG roles, for example, a particular type of senator "Because those who sat back and just watched and observed, but those who wanted to be a leader and wanted to speak did it right away." While youth were given little choice on roles, they were given opportunity on how they would play these roles. Adults did not tell them how they should act during the Assembly; this was theirs to do. "The people who were helping run the programs" were not always around and this "was a good thing because what helped is that they opened it up and let us do it." Another said it this way; "You don't feel like there's an authority in the room. You just feel like you want to go by the rules, because you don't want to cause any problems because then it's just annoying." Having the option to decide how to do the required work was important. "If everybody did nothing and if we just had somebody hand us a bill, it wouldn't be Youth-in-Government."

Because these roles were real for them during Model Assembly, the young people began to realize that their work could be consequential for them; what the experience turned out to be and how it would affect them was up to them. They were the authors of the event's experience and meaning. "We were responsible more for what we wanted to make out of it, like we didn't have an assignment to get finished. We didn't have this to make sure that we were understanding and learning. So that was left up to us to do. So we had to take more responsibility upon ourselves." Young people defined YIG's curriculum as both open and formal, with rules, and also with choices. This is one of the program's strengths and what makes Model Assembly such a powerful experience. On this the official and youth descriptions agree.

Activities

Young people said that YIG activities are required, done individually or in pairs, and occur only during the time they are involved in YIG. Activities are required as part of a larger choreography, joining individual and pairs to delegations and to the whole. There is a great deal of role interdependency, a schedule formalizing these interconnections and sequences. For example, "My job was to write opinions on every upper house bill, which turned out to be about 250 or 300 bills, and review them for constitutionality or clarity, some of the closure lines on how much it would cost, and where the money would come from and then write opinions on them." Talking about their activities, youth spoke of "have to," "supposed to," and "needed to be done," a language of responsibility, typical adult language. For example, one person described her work thus: "I have to write a bill."

These activities were done individually, except for the lawyers who worked in teams, and this was an essential part of their work. One described team activity: "We recognized the tasks that needed to be done, and we worked together and apart and combined our resources and put together a good brief. We had to work fairly independently from everyone else because we couldn't get together a lot obviously."

When Model Assembly ended, so did this work. It was an event, not everyday life. It was citizen play, not ongoing citizen work.

While much here fits with official descriptions, there is incongruence too. They describe most activities as occurring as individual and isolated. Is this really how state government works? In summary, YIG was experienced as powerful by young people because it was an opportunity to try government by being government. During the Model Assembly's four days, the experience was good and meaningful, their work important. When it was over, it just ended, with no possibility of continuing. Where to find opportunities in the everyday to be and to experience oneself as skillful and competent? How to carry on this work after the simulation ended? How to use what was learned in the simulation for self and others everyday? These questions and interests were not voiced by young people in PA or at the YSC.

Young people in the YSC do not talk about their everyday experience in these ways. For them, the YSC initiative is potent precisely because it was not a simulation, it is real life. YSC is a pathway into the real work of the museum, real work with real and profound consequences for them and others.

YOUTH SCIENCE CENTER (YSC)

Young people participating in the Youth Science Center remind program developers and adult staff of the importance of safe and comfortable spaces for young people. This is basic but often forgotten in youth civic engagement conversations.

Aims

Before they are actively involved, many young people say that they come to YSC for a job, because they need money. Others are influenced by friends and family: "My mom made me come" or "My friend just told me about it and he said to call, and I didn't really know anything about it." A third group signs up because of their interests. "I think I needed more stuff to do out of the normal, since [the educational enrichment program] ended, because it was my mainstay of like extra weird stuff to do and I think I needed more of that because it had gotten kind of boring and I was just doing normal school." Yet others simply wanted "something to do." "It's work so I don't sit home for lack of something to do," one young person said. YSC gives me a reason to " . . . leave my house and have somewhere to go right after school. Because I used to come home and just go straight to sleep or whatever and wait until night and then go out," said another. For young people YSC can be employment, something to do, or a way to pursue personal interests. These answers change after the first few weeks at the YSC.

> At first they were all bored when they first came here. They were like, my mom made me come. Everybody's mom makes them come to volunteer at the YSC. Nobody really wants to come. That's work for free. After the first week they didn't know who I was, they were real quiet. By the end of the second week, I'm seeing smiles cracking; I'm seeing work actually get done.

Although young people say they come to YSC for many reasons, they stay because "It is not your typical work place." It is unusual they can "do things." The YSC is also atypical because "Here you can come in late and they'll understand. It's a very understanding, caring environment."

Young people choose to stay at YSC because their experience is special and unique, not otherwise available, and at a place where they feel supported, encouraged, and can contribute to the collective and do public work. For young people the YSC is much more than what is given in the official aims. It is a place of support, encouragement, and opportunity. It offers purpose and a safe space to be who they are and become who they want to be, now and in the future. Young people and their ideas, talents, and contributions are the foci and it is these that are recognized and incorporated into ongoing museum work. It is through them that one gets to science. While all of this work connects with science and science learning, these are not the focus. Young people feel they are the priority.

Strategy

To young people, YSC emphasizes joint work with other young people, adult YSC staff and museum professionals, on teams, doing actual and authentic museum projects requiring their ideas and opinions, not just their bodies and their time. As one said, "We're doing the work as a professor" and not "just teaching assistants." When asked how they get the work done, young people refer to their "project" groups. Here, they meet diverse peers and YSC adult staff, along with professionals from throughout museum departments. "It's just where teenagers, people around my age, go to work with volunteers, work with people that come from all different walks of life. It's way different from school." YSC groups have a dual purpose: they support getting the work done while also making it possible to meet both other youth and adults too.

The work is real for the museum and thus to them; it is neither simulation or made-up work: It is everyday museum work. "The YSC just kind of opened up the door for them, you know, it kind of opens up like, this is the Science Museum, this is what we do and we . . . do different things that you [can] think about." Youth do important projects, authentic work, such as "building stuff upstairs on the third floor (one of the exhibit halls)," "running programs for volunteers, teaching volunteers," and helping the community by providing an "after school program for the kids. So the kids have something to do." To them, the job is unusual because of its demands to quality and the kind and amount of their input—they are encouraged, indeed at times required, to offer suggestions.

To accomplish such real and meaningful work, they must give more than just time, in contrast to their experience on most other volunteer or service-learning projects. Knowledge, ideas, and suggestions too must be given; they must give themselves. "The stuff you say actually has an impact. Cause in school you can say a lot of stuff and they won't pay attention really." The YSC, "It's like overly open." The staff continually asks for young people's ideas, they said.

> [Adult staff person] had been throwing a lot of ideas out there and he said if you happen to think of anything, then say something. And I think he was hoping that out of one of these ideas, concepts of calculus he was throwing out, someone would come up with an idea. So he was just using a lot of different examples.

Because of this "we have a big voice here." Having a voice, completing necessary museum work and doing so with a diverse group of other youth is, in their view, YSC's strategy.

The YSC has obviously succeeded in its strategy of involving young people in real and necessary museum work. This is not a pretend place where the work is simulated, irrelevant, or simple made-up. This is also more than "a job," just doing a task; they can influence, even shape the project's direction and result.

Ethos

"They do a really good job of not treating us like little kids." For most, this sums up what it is like to work at YSC: The place is open, they are asked to be responsible and are respected by adult staff, and learn. And they have fun! These are YSC values, embodied in the adult staff and their practices. YSC is a good place for kids, young people say. Young people most often talk about YSC's "openness." For them this includes having the option of controlling their schedule. "We set our own break time and own hours to come in." Some also choose when to join. "I joined like, yeah, half-way through the season." Everyone talked about having a choice about what work they can do, although this has limits. "When we're in the YSC, we're free to do basically what we feel as long as it's actual work and it's actually helping the YSC succeed in something." The only limit to openness is that how they act has to be "publicly appropriate," which means "dressing right" and completing daily work objectives. This openness allows them to be who they cannot be elsewhere. "I'm allowed to be a little more myself here, because it's more open." At the YSC, young people found a place where they had opportunities and options and this made it possible for them to be themselves in new and competent ways. This is role and self-experimentation, and a test of self-mastery.

This made YSC a special place and experience. They experienced it as a place where they were encouraged and allowed to be who they are and who they wanted to become and be. What prevents them from being themselves elsewhere? Other places are not as open as YSC. Here they can make mistakes and these are used to facilitate learning; they are given the opportunity to take on various activities of interest to them; they are invited and supported in exploring job, self, roles, and relationships, in addition to science.

With these choices comes responsibility. But this is not burdensome; rather it is being treated as a grown up. Being expected to be responsible as persons and as workers is to be taken as a real, that is, adult, person.

> We want responsibility because they're not really there to tell us exactly what we're supposed to do. We pretty much learn. If you decide to come in late, they'll understand sometimes. Well, you can't just stroll in thirty minutes late whenever you feel like it. They're like well . . . we need to work on this. Next time maybe you can call. I don't really know anyone being fired for coming in late cause everybody just learns that the first time.

Having these choices and being asked to be responsible is to be treated and respected as a person. Young people's stories are filled with examples of how adult staff respect them or check on how they feel about how they are being treated.

> I do remember one time we were having this leadership meeting, it was on a leadership Saturday where all the groups come together, and I don't remember her name, but a lady told us we were getting a million dollars donated to the YSC. We were like, oh my gosh! And we were psyched about it. And none of the leaders knew about this, like the older ones. And [staff person] was like, what? Then at the end she's like, well, we're not getting a million dollars, I was just kidding you. And she said, "But those are really good ideas though." Everybody was mad. So the next Wednesday that I came in, [a adult staff person] said something and I was like are you kidding about this too? She was like, "Oh my gosh, we've ruined them, we've lost their trust." They had to have a meeting over that. She puts a lot of care into us. A lot of them care about how we feel. They worry about our feelings and we worry about theirs. If somebody's having a downer day, they'll be like do you want to talk about it?

Being treated with respect and being given so many options reinforced that their work is meaningful. Thus they want to do a good job—one that does not make Youth Science Center or Science Museum of Minnesota "look bad." Yet doing "real work" adds pressure. "Well, like sometimes there is a lot of pressure put on you when you are a leader. When you're a leader, because you are in charge of everything that you have to do." All are asked to take on leader roles and with this comes responsibility and respect, giving added importance to their efforts. This too brings pressure to do the job well. All of this is learning work roles, recognizing that your voice matters and can be heard, mastering group roles—all basic to citizen work.

YSC remains for young people a place of learning and exploration. "The YSC gives people the opportunity to grow. And they're growing, they're learning about something that . . . there's no web page classes in schools, and if there is, it's not fun. I think the whole purpose of the YSC is to have kids learn things while they're having fun." In the end this all adds up to making YSC:

> The most positive place basically. Me being still in high school it's probably the most positive place because there's no negativity flowing around the YSC. You can't be negative. It's a place where

you get paid to have fun or to laugh, to get along with others and learn about others. So why would you ruin that?

Curriculum

Young people help design the YSC curriculum–it is co-created, emergent, and filled with choice, with the work always about science. By science, young people mean investigating and research into both the physical and social worlds (for example, projects in which they taught math, physics, and culture). This science focus is central, shaping YSC's intended outcomes as well as its activities. Here too, the official and youth descriptions match. The young person's voice tells how to make a program inviting, inclusive, and participatory. YSC works because it allows uncertainty and ambiguity to flourish. While the outcome might be named and defined, the process to accomplish this is not; instead it is co-created with staff and emergent. When staff name the work as such, it opens a space for young people to meaningfully contribute and not simple participate in a pre-formed educational program. This ethos provides spirit, direction and substance to the curriculum which is itself a goal and process.

Inside this science focus, the curriculum is emergent, with young people bringing up ideas for inclusion as goals, objectives, practices and steps.

> They let you do like anything, cause you can suggest anything and do anything really. Cause I mean they'd let you go on the computers and find cool stuff and share it and then might even go. Just this last time I was waving the laser in kind of a cool way and it caused a weird-like shape to appear and Bruce was talking about it and they tried to figure out more about it and turned out that we couldn't really do anything cool with it. But we just you know, he just kind of like took that idea, and felt kind of special because he was paying attention to my idea I guess.

Because of this way of working, young people believe that their suggestions are taken as real and may be acted upon and become real. "Mostly like what we want to happen, if we come up with suggestions. [Staff people] are always saying come up and come tell us and we'll develop, try to develop something out of it and we'll be like the leaders."

Young people know that their next idea or focus might come to them at any moment. This belief comes from working with adult staff open to each moment's possibility; they too begin to see in this way, like an infinite, and not finite game (Carse, 1986).

> The whole entire group was sitting around and he was drawing on the board. We were talking about regular polygons. And we worked out way up, we were like what's the world for a hundred-sided polygon? And then we said, "What's the name for an infinite-sided polygon," and it was a circle. And I was just trying to think of what can you take and make it into a triangle and would transform into a circle. And I came back the next day and I said what if we used a laser inside of a circular mirror and just bounce it around in there?

In this we also learn how young people understand curriculum, here, as process, a co-creative process. They do not come to YSC to be taught science, although they say that they learn some of this. Rather they come to YSC to engage science, which to them means "creating" with adult staff. "[Staff] never come in and tell us do this, do that, you do this, you do that. It's never been that way. Everything that happens in the YSC is based on somebody's idea, some younger staff member's idea or a volunteer's idea." Throughout YSC, the idea of choice is central. Its curriculum is filled with choices. Young people choose what to do. "Basically we don't send anyone on their jobs, like you do this, you do that." They also choose how to do it. "They don't tell you every step about how to go about accomplishing [the work]." Finally, they can choose when to do it. "We just ask people what would you like to do, and we sit back and wait for it to happen. So we're just real patient," as long as the focus remains somehow connected to the larger ideas of science. As one young person said, "They do have a plan, and they will stop you from going completely off, but they let you wander quite a bit, I suppose."

Youth descriptions of the curriculum provide additional insights into the official description of the curriculum. While they agree that the curriculum does emerge from young people's questions and the larger concerns and needs of the museum, for young people the focus on science is only part and, for some, a small part of its curriculum. What matters the most to them is its emergent and inclusive atmosphere. This is framed within the ideas of inquiry, invention, and education. These three ideas join to create the curriculum that is animated through collaboration with adult staff and explicit modeling of these by adult staff. Young people engage in activities related to these ideas.

Activities

Young people know they are doing work that is central to the larger museum and to YSC. In activities, they learn and have available new and, they say, unique roles, new ways of being youth. They participate in activities that matter to the larger museum and thus to them. They work in teams and help build and maintain these. "First we have to have team builders, that's the number one thing" as a way to "get them as close as possible working with each other." To another:

> I look at one person really to be the one who's the hardest to work with, the quiet one. He's real reserved, so I try to get him into everything. And once he gets into it and . . . I don't really like to say it, but it's just like they follow. The girls, if I get the joking sister to do it, which is pretty much easy, the older sister will do it–the older sister is the quiet, laughing one.

As team members, they are a resource to the larger museum and help it achieve its overall mission of educating the public, including children, young people, and families, both in the building and in community. "We go to outreach and go to Frog Town and do activities with little kids." Young people are also involved in co-creating exhibits for the several exhibit halls and for conducting supervised field research as well as for working with field artifacts. One young person told about his work in the dinosaur hall, "I kind of missed out on casting so I am molding the casts. Now I have been out just putting the casts together into the real, like, the real skeleton of it." To the youth, these activities provided insights, and real learning, allowing them to take on the roles of leader, teacher, group facilitator, field researcher, and so on–roles that are to them new, unique and challenging; these for them are the opportunities opened up by YSC.

In summary, it is seen that young people's experience of YSC fits well with its own formal description. From their experience, YSC staff and activities do invite and support young people participating in the museum. They experience YSC as a place where they are allowed to do important work for the museum and others (e.g., group, visitors, community members, etc.). It is this direct participation in "real" museum work that makes YSC a meaningful and important place for them.

What their descriptions add to the formal descriptions is an emphasis on creating a comfortable and safe space for their participation. Often this is either presumed or forgotten about in youth civic engagement conversations. Young people talking about the value and importance of the YSC remind us how critical this basic element is to good work with young people.

COMPARING YOUTH DESCRIPTIONS OF YCE PROGRAMS

All three programs show two main similarities from the perspective of young people. First, these programs were unusual in that they provided a unique and alternative experience in their everyday lives. This chapter began with a review of what young people told us was their typical everyday experience–silenced, structured, and supportive. In these youth civic engagement initiatives, they had voice and choice. They had a role in determining the shape of their daily activity and were responsible for realizing the project's ethos. What they did and said mattered to the project, to their work, and also to the group and to the larger community. These programs provided an alternative to their typical silenced everyday life-experience.

All of the programs were focused on encouraging and supporting them in doing something, in part because the projects needed their active participation. This adult need led to youth seeing them as valuable experiences. Young people participated and also got something done. In Public Achievement, this included completing a project, getting along with one's group, and figuring out how to get something done in their school, city, or community. In Youth-in-Government, young people wrote legal briefs for court cases, bills to be debated on in the legislature, stories for the daily newspaper produced over the four weeks, convincing arguments, skillfully fulfilling the role, and making the whole experience safe for participants. Participants in the Youth Science Center talked about teaching science in the community and museum, creating exhibitions, and conducting research. Young people described these programs as spaces in which they did things that mattered not only to their own development and learning, but also to other people and places.

The youth descriptions also highlighted several differences between the programs. These differences show two of the programs as similar–YSC and PA–and one as different–YIG. The traditional way of describing programs, the one we used in the last two chapters, does not illuminate these differences. It is the young people's experience of the initiative and the meaning they attach to their actions within the initiatives that make the differences appear. Young people's experience of the three initiatives are summarized in Table 5.

When it comes to adult involvement, young people in YSC and PA describe an active and involved role of adult as being-with-them, helping them figure out and take action on their projects, but not taking over the project (Zeldin, Camino, & Mook, 2005). In YIG, young people described adults as setting-up the structure and then removing themselves from the simulation. While both created environments for youth participation (Hart, 1992), the differences shed light on adult roles in youth civic engagement programs. Young people said it was valuable to have adults who acted as guides and coaches, helping them reflect on the challenges they encountered, what they were learning, and how they might proceed.

How young people understood their work within each program provides another contrast. In YIG, young people talked about the program as educational. For them, this program taught them something that they would likely use later in life. The content and product of their work was relatively unimportant outside of the program, but their involvement and the process would yield results later on, especially when choosing a career or having a diverse (geographically at least) group of friends. In YSC and PA, young people talked about how their actions mattered right now and how not taking action would have consequences not only for them but for others in their schools, organizations, or communities. They did not talk about the programs as educational but, rather, as supporting their work on issues they cared about. These programs supported young people in doing something for a community of people now and not preparing them for doing this work in the future. It helped them "make a difference." By doing it now, the programs believe young people will be better able to also do similar work in the future. One program

TABLE 5. Summation of Young People's Experience

	YIG	YSC	PA
Power/role legitimacy	Given by adult leaders	Co-created by kids and adults	Youth created around project
Major youth role orientation	Student	Staff	Group member
Context for the activity	Simulated	Real	Real
Citizenship temporal orientation	Later	Now	Now

was framed as preparatory for future action, while the other two framed themselves as supporting learning and action in the here and now.

This framing had important consequences for the young people who participated, with PA and YSC members talking about how they were unlike "students," because they were taking meaningful and consequential action for themselves and for others. These two programs opened up alternative role identities to these youth, who rarely described themselves as being students or even young people. These programs did not remind them that they were students; indeed, they suggested a number of other ways they could understand and describe themselves differently–as teacher, scientist, group leader, staff, group member, contributor to community issues. Young people in YIG never stopped seeing themselves as students. One way to interpret this is that these young people did not experience themselves as citizens. But this is unlikely. They talked about having a real voice and needing to make important choices in ways very similar to young people involved in the other two programs. In YIG, young people act out a role, one that clearly referred to and was understood as being adult–senator, legislator, lawyer. They choose to use this program to explore future and, for many, newly possible careers, but the program did not influence or challenge their contemporary identities. They were still students and young people performing. They were not real roles they could do for real anytime soon. It was something to aspire to; not something they could be or do now outside of the initiative.

COMPARING ACROSS INITIATIVES
AND BETWEEN OFFICIAL AND YOUTH DESCRIPTIONS

Comparing official and youth descriptions of these three initiatives within the analytic categories of aims, strategies, ethos, curriculum, and activities illustrates how these two different perspectives provide new and deeper insight. This challenges the idea that the official description is a full and accurate one. Problems arise when it is these that are used to evaluate and study youth civic engagement. There, adult meaning and concerns are privileged. Making judgments on program improvement and offerings cannot be confidently made without other perspectives, especially those of the participants. Indeed, is not this what the democratic ethos basic to such projects teaches?

How does adding young people's perspectives challenge what should be evaluated and how? Looking at "learning outcomes" and "focus of

TABLE 6. Youth Civic Engagement from Young People's Perspectives

	Description	PA	YSC	YIG
Learning Outcomes	Official	Public Work Citizenship	Science	Government Citizenship
	Youth	How to get something done in a particular context Have and use their voice Work with others		
Practice focus	Official	Getting projects done	Learning about science	A good simulation
	Youth	Being provided with new opportunities and supported to contribute to real and necessary work		

practice" provide useful insights into how the focus and purpose of youth civic engagement programs, evaluation, and research are enriched when other perspectives are included. This is seen in Table 6. Young people across the three initiatives agree on learning outcomes and focus for practice. These differ from official description in both content and form. Young people want more attention given to what they can now do and to the practice they master through participating. These they name and talk about as being useful for many contexts, although their success using these elsewhere depends on the barriers they encounter and the support they receive in those spaces. Emphasized by young people is the opportunity that these initiatives provide for doing real and mean-ingful work. The three initiatives succeeded according to the young people because each respected, valued, and made it possible for them to contribute their talents to the overall work, whether simulation, project, or actual practice. Here are seen new possibilities for programming, for evaluating and for studying youth civic engagement.

REFERENCES

Aitken, S. (2001). Geographies of young people: The morally contested spaces of identity. London: Routledge.

Austin, H., Dwyer, B., & Freebody, P. (2003). Schooling the child: The making of students in classrooms. London: The Falmer Press.

Bennett, S. (1997). Why young Americans hate politics, and what we should do about it. *PS: Political Science and Politics, 30*(1), 47-52.

Butts, R. F. (1980). The revival of civic learning: A rationale for citizenship education in American schools. Bloomington, IN: Phi Delta Kappa Educational Foundation.

Camino, L., & Zeldin, S. (2002). From periphery to center: Pathways for youth civic engagement in the day-to-day life of communities. *Applied Developmental Science,* 6(4), 213-220.

Carse, J. (1986). Finite and infinite games. New York: Free Press.

Frazer, E., & Emler, N. (1997). Participation and citizenship: a new agenda for youth politics research? In J. Bynner, L. Chisholm, & A. Furlong (Eds.), Youth, citizenship and social change in a European context. Aldershot, UK: Ashgate Publishing Company.

Gibson, C. (2001). From inspiration to participation: A review of perspectives on youth civic engagement. New York: Carnegie Corporation of New York.

Hart, R. (1992). Children's participation: From tokenism to citizenship. Florence, Italy: UNICEF International Child Development Centre.

Hildreth, R. (1998). Building worlds, transforming lives, making history: A guide topublic achievement. Minneapolis, MN: The Center for Democracy and Citizenship.

James, A., & James, A. (2004). Constructing childhood: Theory, practice and social policy. New York: Palgrave MacMillan.

Joplin, L. (1995). On defining experiential education. In K. Warren, M. Sakofs, & J. Hunt, Jr. (Eds.), The theory of experiential education. Dubuque, IA: Kendall/Hunt Publishing Company.

Lesko, N. (2001). Act your age! A cultural construction of adolescence. New York: Routledge Falmer.

Prout, A. (2005). The future of childhood. London: RoutledgeFalmer.

Way, N. (1998). Everyday courage: The lives and stories of urban teenagers. New York: New York University Press.

Winter, N. (2003, April 24). Social capital, civic engagement and positive youth development outcomes. Retrieved January 2, 2006, from http://www.policystudies.com/studies/community/Civic%20Engagement.pdf

Zeldin, S., Camino, L., & Mook, C. (2005). The adoption of innovation in youth organizations: Creating the conditions for youth-adult partnerships. *Journal of Community Psychology,* 33(1), 121-135.

Adult Descriptions of Public Achievement

INTRODUCTION

Most youth civic engagement programs, initiatives, or efforts involve adults. Yet, in many studies of youth civic engagement the voices of volunteer adults are left silent. This is expected, given the dominant focus on "measuring" how programs "meet" civic engagement outcomes. When adults are discussed, it is often about how to "train" them better to work with youth. It is important to keep in mind that the role of adults varies according to program type and design–there is no such thing as a youth worker. Adults who work with youth range from credentialed professionals such as teachers and youth workers to volunteers. There will be differences in training and supervision, in curriculum, and desired outcomes. In the last chapter we saw that youth in different programs had different understandings of the roles that adults played in their efforts. In this chapter we consider the perspectives of adults in Public Achievement. Like youth, adult "coaches" (the term PA uses for experiential educators) have vastly different descriptions and understandings of PA than the official literature.

We only examine one program here, because we feel PA is typical of many curricular and extra-curricular youth civic engagement efforts–activities with a curriculum (broadly understood) in which adults *helped* or *facilitated* the efforts of young people to participate in and learn through civic engagement. Like youth, adult PA "coaches" had a different interpretation of what PA was about than the official literature. In this section, we briefly describe adult perspectives on PA within the same categories we used for youth and official programs. The outstanding feature of each description was the tension between what PA was supposed to be like (derived from official program literature, curriculum training, their own ideas) and the reality of trying to work democratically with a group of young people. In the final section, we discuss the way in which this tension eventually became a source of meaning in their work with young people. Table 7 summarizes the adult perspectives.

Most of the adult coaches we interviewed were college students, though some were teachers, Americorps members, or parent or community volunteers. Like youth, only some sought out this experience. Many students signed up for a particular college course and then were surprised to find out that it had PA as a service learning component. All coaches went through an orientation and training that introduced them to the aims, ethos, and strategies of the program. This training introduced coaches to a few key activities intended to orient them to their work with

TABLE 7. Official and Adult Perspectives Compared

Descriptor	Official Program	Adult Perspectives
Aims	Engage young people in doing and learning "public work" and produce changes in communities, broadly defined	Help kids do something Try, but fail to help them learn about citizenship and politics
Strategy	Public work: young people learn about politics and citizenship through the actual experience of productively engaging the public world	Help a group of young people on their project, give structure, guidance, but not direction
Ethos	Public focus Co-creative	Co-creative but youth driven
Curriculum	Green book	Green book, trainings, formal and informal debriefings, six-stage process
Activities	Public work	Weekly meetings, action projects

young people. However, the program was explicit that most of the learning would come "on the job." After each session with young people, coaches would de-brief with professors and teachers to reflect on their experiences with youth. According to the guidebook, these sessions were also supposed to be forums for coaches to reflect on their own development as citizens.

Even though many had not heard of PA before, most were attracted to the official vision and description of PA after orientation. They were attracted to its connection to the civil rights movement, the idea that they are helping young people do something significant, and the hope that public work is possible. As one coach said, "I want people to think about their role in society more. And what citizen means and that we don't live in our own private life. There's a whole society out there that we're a part of that we should care about too, instead of just living in our little lives." Another said that "I hope really to empower the kids, that they're accomplishing things." However, this "ideal" vision of the aim of PA quickly came into conflict with the reality of working with youth. Reflecting on her first day, one coach commented:

> D-Day, I was thinking about all the philosophy we learned, about you know, about these geniuses, you know, [Paulo] Freire, and [Myles] Horton, and all these people and thinking, you know like what would they do. And then the kids come in, and all those theories go out the door and you're left with these kids.

Another coach articulated the sometimes confusing dialectic between ideals and reality in her statement that,

> PA demonstrated to me that my ideal is probably very separated from the reality of this type of work, public work, because you forget about the logistical issues of working with people. And that your passion does not necessarily translate into somebody else's passion. Even the understanding of what needs to be done is so incredibly different. That's just a reality-check portion of it. I think there's also the hopeful portion of it that PA has given to me. I think I would need to do it again to really know how I felt about it for sure.

Here we can see the disjuncture of ideal and reality, of theory and practice, of hope and disappointment that structures the experiences of trying to work democratically with youth.

Adult coaches had a more or less firm grasp of the official ethos of PA, public work. They also understood the "ideal" strategy of co-creating a democratic group that would carry out a project to make a lasting public contribution. They understood that this project would have a series of steps and that through this work their job was to help young people learn about citizenship and politics. However, the prime difficulty was the tension between "letting" their group "drive" and helping the group carry out public work. Or as one coach said, the most difficult thing is "probably trying to find a balance between telling them what to do and letting them choose." Other coaches described this balancing in terms of "push versus pull," "riding a roller coaster," "a juggling act," "spinning plates," and "being kid bumpers on bowling lanes." It is not entirely clear whether this role confusion is a product of poor training or a necessary part of democratic work with youth.

The six-stage process as articulated in the PA guide book did not play out in practice. One coach captured this with her statement that, "Kids don't go by the script. And you're like, why?" When confronted with the situation of being "left with these kids" and not knowing what exactly to do, coaches typically improvised, negotiating in the moment to craft a workable group. This element of reaction and improvisation never went away. Coaches all recalled how their groups could be radically different within a single session and also from week to week: "It's a varied experience, as well, from time to time. There are ups and downs as the group's behavior and enthusiasm dictates [what happens in the group]." All coaches commented on the important skills of observing, listening, and reacting to groups.

While group dynamics were a source of frustration, as the year went on many coaches gradually improved their abilities to read, react, and interact with their groups. In our view, the most effective coaches found a mediated practice that matched their own group, as opposed to "trying out" a new theory or an "all encompassing angle" each week; they became, in Donald Schön's (1983) phrase, "reflective practitioners."

The activities of coaches focused on the weekly meetings with their groups. In this sense, the activities were rather mundane and overwhelming. Coaches were first forced to confront basic group dynamics. One coach commented that "Kids are not used to democratic action. Because my kids will go running around and I have to tell them not to." There were often interpersonal disputes that coaches mediated. The second dominant reality was trying to construct and carry out a project. From deciding what to do and then doing the necessary tasks, the coaching role was very much directed at managing these activities such as figuring out how to motivate students who did not want to be there, how to get permission for public actions, remembering assignments, and keeping records. Given the sometimes overwhelming nature of the weekly meetings and the difficulties of trying to construct a project, coaches did not feel like they were fulfilling their roles as experiential civic educators. They were acutely aware that they were supposed to capture teachable moments and evaluate the group's activities in terms of their political dimensions but commented that they rarely, if ever, actually did these things. This was a source of frustration and contributed to many coaches feeling that they had "failed" to fulfill their role.

COACHING AS A MEANINGFUL EXPERIENCE

Even though many of the comments described above highlight the disjuncture between the theory and practice of PA, a vast majority of coaches came to the conclusion that this was an important and meaningful personal experience. In this section, we will offer coaches' descriptions of the ways in which this experience gave them meaning and became meaningful. During orientation and training, coaches were explicitly instructed that this was not solely a program for youth, but they were supposed to develop as citizens through coaching. However, most individuals we interviewed focused exclusively on their work with young people. In fact, our interviews seemed to be the first time that they had reflected on the meaning for themselves.

One named source or meaning was getting to know and coming to "like" their group. Coaches came to identify with their group, to become emotionally invested in the group's triumphs and disappointments. When asked whether this was a meaningful experience, a coach answered:

> Yeah, it definitely has [been]. I mean I've learned a lot . . . it's been great. Like no matter how much I complain, and how stressful it is, or whatever, like it has been really interesting and a really meaningful experience. There are some kids that I feel really close to. I think that makes it worthwhile, regardless of whether or not we complete our project. It is also meaningful in those moments where we have some sort of breakthrough. Everything about it has been a really nice learning experience. I mean it may not be this pleasant experience, but it has been a really good exercise. It was also my first experience with kids, and that taught me a lot.

The end of this quote points to a second source of meaning–coaches felt they learned through the experience. There were two different levels of learning. On the first level was learning how to perform their role, new skills such as facilitating, listening to students, managing conflicts, planning, evaluating, and the like. Coaches could name these skills, the moments in which they developed them, and some even named instances in which they "tried out" these new skills in other domains of their lives. For instance, one coach told a story about how she interacts differently with her father. Before the course, she and her dad tended to "butt heads a lot" because they had very different political views. Now, she reports using questions to "get my point across, instead of just going up against him."

On the second level, coaches learned a great deal about and from the individual members in their group–what they care about, how they learn, and what their lives are like inside and outside of school. Coaches were reminded of what it was like to be in middle or high school, what the competing pressures were, and how civic engagement was often a low priority. One coach said she learned from her group,

> . . . that they view things differently. Or to see how they do absorb knowledge. It's one of those things that you don't visualize usually, how you learn. So to see little kids learning things for the

first time that you've already learned, it's easier to see the process of how they learn. And then yeah, when they say something that you wouldn't expect them to say because they view the world in such a different way.

Coaches also learned from the young people in their group the promise and excitement of taking action. Many times this involved groups or certain students transcending what the coach thought was possible. One coach said that her group "taught me [about] the things that people can accomplish. Because who would have thought that we could have pulled off a [multi-school] gathering in four weeks. And it could go so well." Others drew inspiration not from accomplishments but from the process of working with youth: A coach commented that meaning came from:

> . . . the feeling of actually contributing and getting kids to think about issues, and I had to dig a little deeper for my group too, cause they chose a topic at first that they didn't really like [Even though students chose their PA issue group, they sometimes did not put much thought into this choice.]. And at the halfway point, it's like, alright what do you want to do, what [bugs] you about this, what would you like to change? Well, what interests you? The war in Iraq. What do you think about it? We don't like it. Go on, I don't like it either. I would get excited, and to see kids get passionate about something that they want to change, that's dangerous. That's what's great.

On a simple level, coaches fed off the students' energy. On another level, coaches were pushed to rethink their ideas about the capacity, agency, and power of young people. In many cases, working with their group invited coaches to re-think their ideas about politics and their own political engagement. One coach commented that,

> I'd say it's given me a sense of hope that I lost for a while, cause it's really easy to become cynical, especially . . . with the whole war and things going on, but it does definitely give you the idea that, well, at least people are trying to make a difference. And that's one [of] the best things that I see, like these are young people that are going to be working towards a future . . .

Even though this coach did not use the language of citizenship, her re-thinking is articulated in the language of hope, of the possibility for people to work together to make a difference in their communities. Here, we can see the ways in which the official program outcome of coaches developing as citizens is being met, albeit in different terms.

CONCLUSIONS

A dominant lived experience of coaching was the disjuncture between theory and practice, between their understanding of what they were supposed to do (according to training and program literature) and then what they actually did. Coaching young people in PA did not follow the prescribed curriculum. Instead it was an emergent process of learning how to work together. We can now see PA from three different perspectives: the official program literature focuses on public work–the co-creation of projects that have lasting civic importance, the young people focus on being able to express themselves and do something to make a difference, and the adult coaches focus on how to work with a group of young people. Neither young people nor adults used the language of citizenship to describe their experiences. They both did, however, describe the ways in which their experiences in PA were personally meaningful. This points to a different way of talking about citizenship not in the language of rights and responsibilities but in the language of the meaningfulness of working with others on public issues.

REFERENCE

Schon, D. (1983). *The reflective practitioner: How professionals think in action.* New York: Basic Books.

The Place of Evaluation

INTRODUCTION

Evaluation is necessary for youth civic engagement (YCE) programs if they are to receive funding and if they want to improve their work. Foundations and other sources have begun to require this as a condition for grants. Scholars and youth advocates have also begun to lobby for evaluation as a way to determine best practices and guidelines for effective programs (Winter, 2003). The result is that there is now a fast growing library of studies of youth civic engagement programs. This chapter examines typical evaluation strategies and compares these to the evaluation we conducted of the three programs, Public Achievement, Youth-in-Government, and Youth Science Center.

Evaluators use a variety of strategies, methods, and techniques to evaluate youth civic engagement programs. They want to know if the initiative achieved the outcome and impact desired by the funding source, scholars, or practitioners. These include improving school performance, increased civic knowledge and skill, development of social responsibility, social and community change, and healthy youth development. In contrast, we sought to understand the program from the points of view and experience of the multiple participants. We had an explicit stance, one which we used to define evaluation and how studies were conceptualized, implemented, and used for understanding and for program improvement. This stance was that much of what goes on in these projects is evaluative in nature (e.g., group reflection) and that program evaluation is a formalization of what occurs in other ways; that this formalization uses a scientific-like method to get at whether an activity works, i.e., accomplishes its goals, does what it says it will do; that there are many alternative designs and methods for doing this rightly and good (for example, by following the American Evaluation Association guidelines for ethical practice); that a primary goal is the use of findings for program improvement (Patten, 1997) and that the involvement of intended users in the study design, implementation, and use is both morally good and politically effective (Fetterman, Kaftarian, & Wandersman, 1996). In these, we chose to work in typical ways. What was different here was not our stance, but how we implemented this.

We wanted to know what they did, how they made sense of it, and what consequences this had for them and others. We did this by asking young people, teachers, youth workers, volunteers, coordinators, principals, parents, and other non-involved young people to teach us as much as possible about the program and about their participation experiences. Both approaches, the typical and ours, shaped the process of evaluation from strategy to design to use of findings for program improvement. Our experience of evaluating these youth civic engagement initiatives suggest an alternative approach and methods for evaluating youth civic engagement programming.

DESIGNING A YCE EVALUATION

Evaluation is a type of research. Unlike other forms, it is concerned with learning if an effort works, and why. "Evaluation is a systematic process for an organization to obtain information on its activities, its impacts, and the effectiveness of its work, so that it can improve its activities and describe its accomplishments" (Mattessich, 2003, p. 3).

This seemingly straightforward and simple activity, concerned merely with describing what programs do, the result of what they do, and making judgment about its accomplishments is actually complex. Because evaluation is a decision-making activity to determine worth or merit (Rossi, Freeman, & Lipsey, 2003), it is more than learning about programs. It also involves deciding if these programs are worthwhile for young people, their communities, and society. These are political concerns requiring a political process. At the center of every evaluation is an important political question: Who gets to define what matters–the questions, the outcomes, and the technical matters, and when?

In youth civic engagement programs, most evaluations are designed by project staff who either hire an evaluator to do the study or do so themselves. They use the project's overall goals to frame the evaluation questions and these, in large part, determine the type of findings that will result, if not the actual results. Table 8 illustrates these issues for the four youth civic engagement approaches described by Gibson (2001). These are pure types, clear in the abstract but at times less so in practice, where there may be elements of one or more approaches and evaluation strategies.

TABLE 8. Defining What Matters

Approach	Goals	Evaluation Questions	Findings
Civic Education	Civic literacy	What did young people learn? How do they make sense of what they learned? What consequence does that have for them and others?	Civic knowledge, skills, and attitudes
Service-learning	Social responsibility	Did this activity benefit their school performance? What do young people now know that they didn't know before? Have young people changed?	Developed sense of social responsibility Ongoing commitment to community service
Social Organizing	Social and community change	What did they do? Did they bring about the change they were seeking? What other unintentional changes did they bring about?	Social change
Youth Development	Healthy young people	What did they do? Are they different as a result of participating? What can they now do that they couldn't do before participating?	Competence Contribution Character Confidence Connections

Table 8 shows how the evaluations of youth civic engagement programs are typically designed. Civic education is an example. The goal is civic literacy and the outcomes are "the knowledge and skills to act as competent citizens" (Milner, 2002, p. 3). Information is collected from young people on the extent to which this knowledge and skill was learned. Success here is when youth remember these well after they leave the program. In contrast, service-learning begins with a very different goal: social responsibility. This shapes what evaluation questions are asked and what information is collected and how it will be interpreted. This same analysis can be done for the other two. Each programmatic offering has built-in goals, which lead to questions, which lead to ways of analysis and to what to look for. Evaluations based on this model are driven by the language and ideas of programmatic designers, not necessarily by young people. Our evaluation took a different approach.

Over the six years that we collected evaluation data, we used two distinct and complementary evaluation orientations: processes and outcomes. Our process evaluation (Patton, 1997) was focused on program fidelity and implementation, looking always at how the program idea and derivative model were implemented and how this could be improved at particular sites and across program locations. Our outcome evaluation strategy, following Patton (1997), also was designed for program improvement. We anticipated that both evaluation strategies would produce information that could be used in the three classical ways: conceptionally, programmatically, and in decision-making (Patton, 1997).

Five questions guided our evaluation design and how it was implemented:

1. What does this project say it is about?
2. How is it organized and carried out?
3. What are young people doing in the program? (Are they doing what they have not done before?)
4. What meaning do they give to their work?
5. What consequences does this work have for them, others, the larger community?

Our evaluation started from the same place as others and then moved in a different direction, given our goals of examining program implementation and program improvement. What was different about our study was that we worked as if we did not understand what anyone was telling us. For example, when a young person said the word "citizenship," we assumed that we did not understand what he or she meant. This strategy opened the door to a deeper interrogation of the insider's experience and brought us to the many ways these projects are experienced and understood by different types of participants–young people, adult coaches, school principals, community leaders, teachers, group leaders, and by different individuals. This gave us a look at what was meaningful to them, as well as to what was done in the program and why.

CONDUCTING A YCE EVALUATION

Evaluations conducted based on the typical approaches to YCE have several commonalties. Most of the time, they focus attention on young people and their behavior. The information they collect refers to individual knowledge, skills, and attitudes. It is the young person who remains the focus of attention and through studying them evaluators learn about these particular youth and programs. How did this program affect this young person's behavior, knowledge and skills? Put another way, the unit of analysis remains the young person. Most evaluations define programmatic results as individual change, even when the program supports young people working in groups. The young person is understood to exist outside of a context–group, program, neighborhood. What is studied is the young person, not the program as such.

Information on individual change is then compared to existing criteria to determine if and to what extent the program reached its goals. It is important to compare the data to expectations (Weiss, 1998). Most often these expectations come from outside of the evaluation, either through other research or by looking simply at the official description of the program. Early chapters in this volume have already made clear the limitations of using expectations such as these for program evaluation. They are only one set of possible program results. Too often, voices of other stakeholders, most critically the participants themselves, are excluded. We believed that we had to learn the expectations of other stakeholders.

These expectations of outcomes we clarified in our evaluations (Hildreth, Baizerman, & VeLure Roholt, 2001). Thus we started with the basic question, "What do you do here?" "What was it like to be you and be in this program?" Rather than import categories and definitions, we hoped to develop rich descriptions of the program. With this data, it became possible to broaden the notion of program results (outputs and outcomes) and, we believe, enrich judgments about program vitality. Thus, when we asked a student what they could do better now than before this program, they might reply "make a phone call." From an adult perspective, this appears to be a normal, common, everyday activity. But to youth, these moments were anything but small, common and normal. We would explore *with* the young person what making this phone call meant for them and their work. They talked about these moments as involving a great deal of group planning and individual courage. Often they celebrated after making the call. This was a difficult and challenging act! A telephone call was not a telephone call but a "telephone call"; for them it was being a courageous citizen and responsible group member. We learned that many seemingly mundane tasks were central elements in developing young peoples' sense of political efficacy. Our openness to young peoples' lived experiences would not dismiss this or the numerous other choices and actions they made and took, as a non-important or non-civic.

Going back and looking at earlier descriptions of the programs, we can understand for evaluation purposes the importance of learning the official descriptions of the program and those of the youth participants. Official expectations include fairly traditional ideas about education and learning while, for youth, their expectations were on how they were viewed by adults and what opportunities they had to participate within the program. They said that successful programs were those in which they had voice and choice. Such information typically is not collected when the focus is on learning civic knowledge, skills, and attitudes. Including the expectations of a wider range of stakeholders is basic to good program evaluation theory and practice (Mattessich, 2003; Patton, 1997; Weiss, 1998), and this is what we included.

Our interest in learning the point-of-view and understanding of multiple types of participants–not simply their behavior–resulted in an alternative conception and approach of what was to be evaluated and, in a larger way, what it means to evaluate youth civic engagement projects. We begin with the latter. Evaluation has to be designed and carried out to fit the context, for it is always a contextualized activity (Mark, Henry, & Julnes, 2000). Because a goal of youth civic engagement is to enhance democratic skills and knowledge and social responsibility, we wanted the evaluation to be democratic in conception and implementation. We designed the evaluation to meet the democratic requirements of inclusion, dialogue, and deliberation (House & Howe, 2000). More importantly, we involved young people in the ongoing design and implementation of the evaluation as one way of ensuring that our evaluation remained democratic.

A democratic evaluation must include the insights and perspectives of all relevant stakeholders (inclusion), not only the most powerful, e.g., funders, program staff, or other adults (House & Howe, 2000), especially when program improvement is a goal (Compton, Baizerman, & Stockdale, 2002). Our evaluation design and implementation included many types of stakeholders in the design, data collection (both as respondents and as evaluators), analysis, and construction of findings, including young people in groups, teachers (when at schools) who were both directly, indirectly, or not at all involved in the program, group facilitators (of all ages), program site coordinators and group facilitator coordinators, agency executive directors and school principals, and other site staff. The actual evaluation interview questions were developed in collaboration with program staff and field-tested with young people who provided us with insightful feedback about how to ask questions and what questions they thought would work the best. In this way, the evaluation reflected the many types of participants and their interests, concerns and ways of understanding. Especially crucial, all interviews were carried out to accomplish two tasks: collect information and learn what this information meant to those involved. As evaluators, we had to learn the many different languages of each project–student, youth, citizen, teacher, program staff, and so on and learn how to accurately grasp the speakers' meanings. When done well, the interviews were more conversation-like and less a formal interview. By working with this intent and gaze we learned what it was like and what it meant to be a participant in these projects.

This dialogic and conversational process of collecting information–learning about the program and participant experience–carried over into data analysis. Typically, we discussed the things we learned (findings) with those who taught us (the interviewees) and with other program staff to get feedback about whether we got it and their take on the meaning and importance of what we learned. We sought confirmation (did we get it right?) or an alternative interpretation (try thinking about it this way). Our initial findings and conclusions were often refined. Many who helped us in these ways also learned about their project as well as ways of thinking and talking about their work as they joined us in this deliberate process of data analysis and interpretation. Each yearly evaluation report (Hildreth, Baizerman, & VeLure Roholt, 2001; VeLure Roholt, Hildreth, & Baizerman, 2003) provided evidence for what we learned, insights, and our recommendations for program improvement, and was used by participants to deepen their own reflection and under-standing of their actions, experiences and the meaning of these.

For example, we often brought back the data we collected to the participants themselves for consideration or reviewed what we had learned with them at the end of an interview. By doing so, they began to see how much work they had accomplished, even if their project had not been finished. Often, this was the first time someone had "reflected" with them about the progress they had made toward accomplishing their goals and completing their action plan. While they were in the middle of the work, they did not recognize or name the numerous contacts they made to learn about their project, the large number of decisions the group made collectively, the research they conducted, and the discovery of dead ends as accomplishments. It was just what they did each week in this group. Discussing the data we had collected with them allowed both them and us to learn how much progress had been done that neither they nor others involved in the program named as accomplishments.

Working in this way, several assumptions underlying each program were made explicit and then interrogated. For example, early-on in the evaluation several young people and program staff asked whether individual skill and knowledge mastery really matter to the project, to themselves and to funders. As they read the evaluation reports and reflected on our interview conversation, they saw a lack of fit between what was learned in the evaluation and how the group process was carried out. Individual improvement or even mastery of civic knowledge, skills, and attitudes did not necessarily lead to a more successful group project. What mattered was the mix of knowledge and skill in the group and members willingness to listen and learn from others. An individual's mastery of civic knowledge and skill came to be seen as less important to members and project staff than being willing to share one's talents and to appreciate the talents of the other group members. An open and inclusive deliberation of evaluation findings with various stakeholders allowed this issue to be considered and discussed and served to problematize major project goals for program designers, staff, funding staff, and young people.

Another rationale for using a democratic approach to evaluating youth civic engagement initiatives is that projects often succeed when young people learn how to evaluate their own actions and use this learning in their ongoing project work. Our approach quickly became a new method of learning for them and for their group, evaluation capacity building (Compton, Baizerman, & Stockdale, 2002), with more aware, insightful, analytic and articulate participants–youth and adults alike.

In this way, we expanded the role of program evaluator to include evaluation educator. We worked explicitly to enhance everyone's understanding of program evaluation as an approach to reflection. This was skill development. The goal was that evaluation "becomes a regular, ongoing practice" (Compton, Baizerman, & Stockdale, 2002). Over the six years of conducting evaluations on youth civic engagement initiatives, our work came to include many activities not typically associated with program evaluators and evaluation (Compton, Baizerman, & Stockdale, 2002). At least once a year we developed and offered training on evaluation theory and practice for program staff and youth participants. These trainings often served the dual purposes of increasing participant's capacity to use and conduct evaluation while also providing a unique context within which we discussed and deliberated with stakeholders on our evaluation and how it could be improved so as to be helpful to them in their everyday project work.

During site visits, we often spent time helping young people create an evaluation for the group's work that could be implemented and later shown to us. At the Youth Science Center, we co-created a mini-evaluation to assess the different ways of engaging visitors. The group brainstormed about different approaches they might use. Over the course of a week, each participant modeled their interactions with visitors on one of these approaches and wrote down what happened when they did. By the end, the group had discovered that one of the approaches seemed to work the best with most visitors. In another example, data were analyzed in a fully transparent process, with stakeholders asked to read the information we collected and make sense of it. It was during these conversations that insights emerged and our democratic approach was institutionalized as a norm of democratic evaluation practice. Finally, we worked with youth and program staff on how to use the evaluation, helped by designing for their use handbooks, worksheets, and other aids for different evaluation stakeholders. All of this was "intentional work to continuously create and sustain overall organizational processes that make quality evaluation and its uses routine," or what Compton, Baizerman, and Stockdale (2002) call evaluation capacity building. But there was more.

Evaluating youth civic engagement programs require consideration of the evaluator as a political actor and the political aspects of evaluation. As evaluators we recognized our political power and responsibilities to those providing funding, participants, and to scholarship. We used this to frame the evaluation strategy and methods. Our actions and activity were continually reflected on to see if we indeed were listening to and involving even the most seemingly powerless participants. Working like this reinforced the political message of power.

Evaluation design and implementation is not only from a book. Many decisions must be made regarding approach, strategy, and methods. There are multiple possibilities for these. The way we conducted our evaluation made these choices transparent and part of our conversations with young people and adults. Their voices were included. We were experts who knew best how to solicit and use their expertise.

This way of working resulted in describing and illuminating project outcomes neither expected nor in the frame of civic knowledge, skills, and attitudes, as typically used. These included knowing how to get something done within a particular context, using one's voice, and taking a political stance on issues they find important but which adults often discount as simplistic or unimportant. Young people taught us that these programs were more than learning civic information and acting like a citizen. Rather, youth civic engagement is about personal meaning and personal public action. For them (and us), YCE is young people doing citizen, i.e., citizenship actions; deciding and choosing in democratic ways–living as citizens! Our evaluation sought to understand if and to what extent these projects supported young people becoming the civic persons they knew themselves to be.

USING YCE EVALUATION

Evaluations of YCE programs include and go beyond the conceptual, programmatic, and decision-making uses of evaluation. Without question, conducting an evaluation should provide information about what goes on in the program (activities, roles, and strategies) and allow program staff and participants to gain a better understanding of the program itself (what they did, how they did it, and alternative ways to name and describe all of this), how the program can be improved, and whether or not it should continue. Evaluation of these programs should also be democratizing (Mathison, 2000).

Evaluations provide a unique opportunity to participate in thoughtful conversations about the purpose and intended results of programs. Citizen action and a democratic process is supported by offering an inclusive invitation to people connected to and participating in the program to also be involved in the evaluation. Evaluation can become more than merely a process that collects data and judges based on external expectations. Instead, it should and can become a space for people concerned about an issue, a program, and in particular young people to be in conversation about all of this and also about what they want for their communities and the young people who live there. By doing so, evaluation is integrated into a youth civic engagement process. Evaluation thus can contribute to the creation and sustentation of democratic space and democratic work.

REFERENCES

Compton, D., Baizerman, M., & Stockdill, S. (2002). The art, craft, and science of evaluation capacity building. *New Directions for Evaluation, 93.*

Fetterman, D., Kaftarian, S. J., & Wandersman, A. (1996). *Empowerment evaluation: Knowledge and tools for self-assessment and accountability.* Thousand Oaks, CA: Sage.

Gibson, C. (2001). *From inspiration to participation: A review of perspectives on youth civic engagement.* New York: Carnegie Corporation of New York.

Hildreth, R., Baizerman, M., & VeLure Roholt, R. (2001). *Major findings year 2 of public achievement evaluation.* Retrieved April 27, 2007, from http://www.publicachievement.org/pdf/evaluations/report2000-1.pdf

House, E., & Howe, K. (2000). Deliberative democratic evaluation. *New Directions for Evaluation, 85*, 3-12.

Mark, M., Henry, G., & Julnes, G. (2000). *Evaluation: An integrated framework for understanding, guiding, and improving policies and programs.* San Francisco: Jossey-Bass.

Mathison, S. (2000). Promoting democracy through evaluation. In D. Hursch & E. W. Ross (Eds.), *Democratic social education: Social studies for social change.* New York: Falmer Press.

Mattessich, P. (2003). *The manager's guide to program evaluation: Planning, contracting, and managing for useful results.* St. Paul, MN: Wilder Publishing Center.

Milner, H. (2002). *Civic literacy: How informed citizens make democracy work.* Hanover, NH: University Press of New England.

Patton, M. Q. (1997). *Utilization-focused evaluation: The new century text (3rd edition).* Thousand Oaks, CA: Sage Publications.

Rossi, P., Freedman, H., & Lipsey, M. (2003). *Evaluation: A systematic approach.* Thousand Oaks, CA: Sage Publications, Inc.

VeLure Roholt, R., Hildreth, R., & Baizerman, M. (2003). *Year four evaluation of Public Achievement: Examining young people's experiences or Public Achievement.* Retrieved April 27, 2007, from http://www.publicachievement.org/pdf/evaluations/report2002-03.pdf

Weiss, C. (1998). *Evaluation (2nd Edition).* Upper Saddle River, NJ: Prentice Hall.

Winter, N. (2003, April 24). *Social capital, civic engagement and positive youth development* outcomes. Retrieved January 2, 2006, from http://www.policystudies.com/studies/community/Civic%20Engagement.pdf

Essential Orientations and Practices

INTRODUCTION

Here we use the official, youth, and adult descriptions of Public Achievement, Youth-in-Government, and the Youth Science Center to get at the essential orientations and practices within all three initiatives. We begin with a description of the ways youth workers can invite, support, and encourage young people's civic engagement. Youth workers have orientations to their work and meaning structures to interpret actions (this kid is acting like a jerk vs. this kid is making a political statement). Practices are the usual or customary ways of performing the youth worker role. Nine convergent themes emerged.

Co-Creation: This Work Is Done with Others, Mostly in Groups, and Relies on Collaboration and Negotiation

Co-creation is an orientation similar to other notions in youth participation (Hart, 1992), youth activism (Ginwright, Noguera, & Cammarota, 2006), and youth/adult partnerships (Camino, 2005; Zeldin, Camino, & Mook, 2005), yet with important differences. Youth participation as an orientation to work with young people remains embedded in an adolescent development frame (Hart, 1992), while co-creation as an orientation is embedded in the human science and phenomenological philosophy. Here young people are not seen in developmental terms but as living in particular life-worlds (Merleau-Ponty, 1962) that shape how they understand and make sense of themselves, others, space, and time (van Manen, 1990). An orientation to co-creation assumes that young people often understand differently the world they share with adults. Co-creating begins by first learning from the young person who they are, not by assuming one knows them because they fit a psychobiological (age) profile.

Youth activism has a different way of understanding young people: as political actors. This fits well the notion of co-creation. Youth activism typically is a moral praxis such as young people taking action against social injustice (Ginwright, Noguera, & Cammarota, 2006). Yet this orientation does not fully capture what we found. Co-creation is not concerned about what issue the group decides to work on but how this work is done. What happens when the young person in front of you is not necessarily concerned about issues of social justice? Must she have a personal concern or stake in a public issue that someone else sees as social injustice? We are after another point: co-creation is about "working together," not about a particular moral agenda. Democratic politics is not necessarily only about responding to social injustice. It is also about working on a whole array of issues. Co-creation is focused on creating a safe and comfortable space for young people to discuss their concerns and talents, listen to others, and decide together if they want to "work on this issue" and, if so, to what end and how?

Youth-adult partnerships (YAP) focus on mutual listening, and thus it may be hard to see a difference between what we call co-creation and the general scholarship on YAP. Both aim to encourage and support "mutuality in teaching and learning between youth and adults as well as mutuality in decision-making" (Camino, 2005, p. 75), differing in degree of required equality in role and responsibility (Camino, 2005; Zeldin, Camino, & Mook, 2005). Co-creation neither encourages adults to get out of the way or remain in control of the joint work. Rather, the adult observes and intentionally and selectively responds to the young people working in the group. Adults may allow most of the important decisions to be made by young people because they want this or they may provide greater scaffolding and even education to ensure that young people are fully informed about situational influences and actors that can either hinder or support their work. These are two of the many options, as seen in the classic "ladder of participation" (Hart, 1992). Co-creation works to situate the work and encourage young people to contribute their individual talent to the group. Basic here is negotiation and politics between and among participants on most topics, from what issue to work on to how to work together. Working together means collaborating and negotiating becomes "how we do things in our group."

Contributory: The Group Works on Real Issues and Addresses Real Concerns and Problems

The work is not simulated. Young people are invited and supported to work on authentic and meaningful projects that have benefits and consequences to themselves and others. The orientation is not to make the work easier or directed to certain outcomes (Moon, 2004) but to support and encourage young peoples' participation in direct practice on issues that others, young people and adults, care about and are involved in. This often means that the initiative must provide the necessary scaffolds (Rogoff, 1990) to ensure that young people's participation is authentic and not contrived or make-believe. Young people do not participate in youth-like ways but by taking responsibility for figuring out, with others, what to do next and then making decisions and taking action. They participate as citizens.

Common to these initiatives is their commitment to inviting and supporting these values and orientations. "Youth can surmount great odds and make significant contributions, but it is not reasonable to expect them to become civically engaged in communities and societies that fail to support them" (Yates & Youniss, 1999, p. 273). The orientation is to support young people in making the contributions they want and can try to make. This requires young people to be informed about useful and appropriate practices specific to issues and contexts. For example, they need to know about likely steps required for their project to be successful. With new information and new understanding of what they could do next, young people are invited and supported in deciding what they will do.

Interrogatory: Questions Initiate and Propel the Project. The Work Is Based on Questions Young People Ask and Is Shaped by Questions They Encounter

These initiatives begin and are sustained by questions, not answers. Inviting or awakening a sense of wonder in young people about an issue or concern is often an important beginning. Assumed is that young people have questions they want to ask and will work at finding an answer when supported and encouraged in doing so. Supporting a general sense of wonder is found in asking questions to open up group time/space for reflection, analysis, and planning. The practice is filled with "good" and "right" questions. Good questions are genuine; they are both open and have some focus (Burbules, 1993). Asking open questions is a commonly taught skill. Our use of the idea involves more than simply asking a question that calls for more than a yes or no answer. In civic youth work, questions serve to direct attention to the world as it is and to the world as it might be. Indeed, the youth worker is an embodied interrogatory about personal and world possibility.

The questions asked by civic youth workers do not have apparent answers; the answer is truly unsettled. Others may have tried to answer questions like those this group is struggling with, but these young people, here and now, do not have an answer. While the openness of the questions make them authentic, good and right questions are also focused; they can be responded to (Burbules, 1993). Asking good and right questions is a skill that invites the group to work at their project with a new or enriched perspective.

Contextual: Activity and Learning Is Contextual. Groups Do Specific, Appropriate, and Necessary Work as Understood and Defined Within a Particular Place, Organization, Neighborhood and Issue

The orientation is toward getting something done, around here, now, while ensuring the actions taken are non-violent, equitable, just and legal. As such, the experience supports–and when successful–teaches group members how to work within a specific and actual space, whether a school, museum or neighborhood. Paying attention to the immediate context supports young people in doing real and meaningful work.

In these initiatives, young people did not work only to their own benefit. While they may have received some reward, their overall aim was to accomplish work seen necessary in the particular context. This serves to keep everything real.

Caring for the World: It Is Presumed that Young People Have a Compelling Care for the World. They Are Not Apathetic or Disengaged, but Care About Public Issues and Problems

Youth civic engagement initiatives often propose they will help young people become engaged. The orientation in these initiatives is based in the assumption that young people are already interested and concerned–about their local community, school, museum, etc. They begin by asking, "What do you care about?" not "Do you even care?" Youth civic engagement initiatives often say they are fighting against youth apathy. From our study, we understand apathy as neutral; it does not mean they are engaged nor does it necessarily mean they are disengaged. In our conversations with young people, they talked at length about the issues and problems they care about. These programs were simply their first opportunity to actually put their care into practice. Civic youth workers create the opportunities for young people to create a personal and collective way of life caring for others in our joint world.

Processual: Like Good Democracies, the Work Never Ends

A common theme across the three initiatives is that a basic outcome is the process. Emphasis is on working with young people to co-sustain an ongoing democratic process in which they are an active and willing part. It is not working toward a pre-determined outcome (Jeffs & Smith, 1999). The civic youth worker does not bring the group his, hers, or someone else's desired outcome. Results come from the work and cannot be known before the work begins. This makes both funding and outcome evaluation difficult, because the group's topical outcomes cannot be known before the group has formed and can change as the group meets and works on their project. Civic youth work is an infinite game (Carse, 1986). It is one that can be continually played because the rules and outcomes are co-created by the work itself, bounded by the core values of democratic, inclusive, just, non-violent and equitable joint work.

Open: The Work Can Be Done in Multiple Ways; the Project Can Often Have Different Foci, and Young People Are Not Known Until They Are Met by Their Work in the Group

Orienting toward openness is important. In these initiatives, this meant that the group decided how they would work together, what they would do to complete the project, and often what issue the group will address. Openness included having methods and process for learning about each other so that each group member came to be seen as an individual who could contribute. Who they are in school, family, neighborhood, and with friends is not who they have to be in the group. Here they could be the person they always wanted to be and was supported to be. Taking on new group roles facilitates this exploration and mastery.

Invitational: Participation and Involvement Is Chosen and Voluntary at the Beginning and Each Time the Group Meets

There are no required activities. Instead, young people choose and un-choose to participate. As the work progresses, young people are continually invited to continue. It is never assumed they have to stay in the group. Civic youth work is based in the belief and fact that young people have much to offer and in our society must be invited to make a contribution. We cannot expect young people to make a public contribution unless there are the necessary opportunities and supports (Yates & Youniss, 1999). Each of these initiatives had an invitational ethos. They recognized young people as having important ideas and novel solutions. They treated young people as responsible and capable of choosing to participate in work they found satisfying and meaningful. Like the civic youth worker, these initiatives embody the invitation to come and try.

To More than Self: The Work Is Always Directed Toward Others and Improving or Making a Difference with Larger Worlds

The orientation is toward doing something for others and getting something done that matters to others. These initiatives are not solely about individual development. The work is directed toward public work (Boyte, 2004), social justice (Ginwright, Noguera, & Cammarota, 2006), creating better communities (Henderson, 1995), community development

(Mullahey, Susskind, & Checkoway, 1999), creating better cities (Chawla, 2003), community service (Radest, 1993), or simply " making a difference." Understood is that working on these activities in these ways has reciprocal benefits that can be described in youth development and educational terms, but this is never the overall aim. Instead, these initiatives value and support young people making a contribution to the ongoing crafting and constructing of their own and larger worlds.

FROM ORIENTATIONS TO PRACTICE TO THEORY

These nine orientations describe the general stance of the work of the three initiatives. These are what participants, adult and youth, said was necessary for the initiative to be meaningful and important to them and the larger community. In the next chapters we re-examine these programs through four different theoretical frames: educational, political, vocational, and youth. All of this is then brought together in the final chapter of the book when we describe civic youth work.

REFERENCES

Boyte, H. (2004). The necessity of politics. *Journal of Public Affairs, 7*(1), 75-85.

Burbules, N. (1993). *Dialogue in teaching: Theory and practice.* New York: Teachers College Press.

Camino, L. (2005). Pitfalls and promising practices of youth-adult partnerships: An evaluator's reflections. *Journal of Community Psychology, 33*(1), 75-85.

Carse, J. (1986). *Finite and infinite games.* New York: Free Press.

Chawla, L. (2003). *Growing up in an urbanizing world.* London: UNESCO Publishing.

Henderson, P. (Ed.) (1995). *Children and communities.* London: Pluto Press.

Jeffs, T., & Smith, M. (1999). *Informal education: Conversation, democracy and learning.* Derbyshire, UK: Education Now Publishing Co-operative Limited.

Ginwright, S., Noguera, P., & Cammarota, J. (Eds.) (2006). *Beyond resistance: Youth activism and community change.* New York: Routledge.

Hart, R. (1992). *Children's participation: From tokenism to citizenship.* Florence, Italy: UNICEF International Child Development Centre.

Merleau-Ponty, M. (1962). *Phenomenology of perception.* London: Routledge.

Moon, J. (2004). *A handbook of reflective and experiential learning: Theory and practice.* London: RoutledgeFarmer.

Mullahey, R., Susskind, Y., & Checkoway, B. (1999, June). *Youth participation in community planning* (Planning Advisory Service Report Number 486). Chicago, IL: American Planning Association.

Radest, H. (1993). *Community service: Encounter with strangers.* Westport, CT: Praeger.

Rogoff, B. (1990). *Apprenticeship in thinking: Cognitive development in social context.* New York: Oxford University Press.

Yates, M., & Youniss, J. (1999). *Roots of civic identity: International perspectives on community service and activism in youth.* Cambridge, UK: Cambridge University Press.

van Manen, M. (1990). *Researching lived experience: Human science for an action sensitive pedagogy.* Ontario, Canada: The Althouse Press.

Zeldin, S., Camino, L., & Mook, C. (2005). The adoption of innovation in youth organizations: Creating the conditions for youth-adult partnerships. *Journal of Community Psychology, 33*(1), 121-135.

Learning and Youth Civic Engagement

In their official descriptions, the Youth Science Center (YSC), Public Achievement (PA), and Youth-in-Government (YIG) say they are practicing experiential education. Young people say their initiative offers rich experience: What does this have to do with civic engagement? It is clear that civic engagement is learning about the *everyday work of democracy* and how to do this, not simply learning *about* democratic citizenship or the citizen role: it is learning experientially–learning the real and the practical. Guided by young people's stories, we describe how this learning works. Then we use our reading of experiential education theory for insights into how each initiative makes the learning in civic engagement real and practical.

READING LEARNING
THROUGH YOUTH CIVIC ENGAGEMENT

Young people said that they were invited to do work together on something that was to them worthwhile and meaningful; this they did, supported by adults. They learned real world knowledge, skills, and attitudes. They learned by engaging new and, at times, challenging activities, people, and ideas. The very act of being involved in new and strange environments and participating in new activities with new people stimulated their work and their reflection on it. When it was guided and a formal part of the work, this reflection could be evaluative, critical, and analytic about self, others, ideas and their work together, thus helping to integrate one's learning into more complex knowledge and a more complex self. All of this came together in the work, in "getting stuff done." Because their accomplishments had public outcomes and uses, the work was significant to the young people. In these moral and psychological universes, youth compared their achievements to those of adults; they were not kids doing kid work but citizens doing the work of democracy. They learned by doing and they learned by reflecting on their work. This is the core of experiential education.

By Offering Invitation

To youth, these initiatives were invitations to naming and acting on what matters to them, an issue they cared about, or a project that could have some impact. Also crucial, young people in each program realized that the work, the project, was theirs and that they had control over what they did, including how they responded to emergent issues, tasks, problems and the rest. In PA, no one took over their project; instead they were invited by their coach to figure out how to get the work done. While many teams did finish their projects, most did not, yet all recognized that they had been offered the unique invitation to try. To youth in YSC, they were invited to play important roles in the museum by helping the museum get its work done. They were expected to contribute directly to the work of the museum, and this produced a bit of anxiety because YSC staff asked them to come up with real-world ideas, ways of making these real, and of presenting what they created to museum officials and visitors.

In YIG, youth said they were invited to run the Model Assembly; they "owned" this weekend. They had to write their own legislative bills, legal briefs, or newspaper articles and these became the focus of meetings; it was this that made their work important. What and how well they produced products directly determined how the Model Assembly would turn out. Young people felt personal responsibility for this event. They were invited to produce this day. They were assumed to be capable, responsible, skillful, and smart. With minor variation, especially in skills and knowledge, the same holds true for PA and YSC. Unlike high school where they are most often bored, passive learners and see teachers seeing them as uninterested, empty vessels to be filled with "knowledge," in these initiatives they experienced an invitation to participate as competent–that they could get it and do the work. Even better, this was the work they were interested in, even cared about.

By Supporting the Work of Democracy

These programmatic invitations only began the learning process and would have been meaningless to them if the adults in the projects did not support them and their work. Youth were provided with different kinds of "scaffolding," structures and process that allowed them to do more than they were capable of doing on their own (Rogoff, 1990). In PA, these were their issue focused groups and a "coach." They soon learned the value of their group. "If you work together, like as a group, you can get things done like really fast." Together they learned that the work could get done and how to do this. If the group got stuck, they could also ask the coach for help. It was the coach who often facilitated initial meetings and helped the group decide on what to do and how to do it.

> Yeah, well, he's like, he doesn't try and be like the leader, or the head guy, he makes us like try and be that or one of us steps up in the day and it works out usually. But sometimes it happens, he has to be it because we don't want to be on task and we need to be because like we might have a guy coming to interview or something.

The coach in the group helped the members recognize that they might be able to get the project done and provided encouragement and support for the group as it figured out what was necessary to get their work done. To youth in YSC, the staff and groups provided similar support.

> When everybody has a different personality, I think you get more work done really. Nobody's a yes man, nobody's thinking the same thing, everybody's using their beliefs and their personal opinions to help build something. And most of the time when we start on something we get finished. I don't know anything that we have not decided all to do that has not been finished in the YSC.

Young people attribute much of what they as individuals accomplished to these groups. And they get so much done because of how adult staff worked with them. Staff did not tell young people what to do; instead, they encouraged and consulted on the group and individual work. "It's like a youth-run environment. It's practically run by youth. But we just have people to help us through things that we can't handle by ourselves." Staff step in and out of the work as needed.

> They encourage. They give comments, compliments. Anything that they feel needs to be done in order for your team or us individually to succeed on something. That's what they do. That's what they feel they have to do. So if they decide to tell us you might want to change that around, it seems like too much, it might not be able to be done on time . . . you hear that a lot, and most people— some people, like me, I don't listen. My stuff is always finished on time. That's just their comments. They never control you and say you can't do this 'cause you know it won't be done on time.

To young people their success in YSC comes from their group and the staff who are constantly present–there to talk with and ask advice.

YIG differs from these other civic education initiatives in the type of adult and programmatic support it provides its young people. Here, youth are given prescribed roles and responsibilities and these are reinforced by veteran participants who offer advice to new members on how to get the work done. Delegation Advisors instruct and give feedback before the Model Assembly. Young people in YIG are guided on what to do and how to do it.

When we first joined Youth-in-Government there was this–I don't know the date–but we went to this meeting where you got all your papers telling you what was in store–number one, what your case was, it gave you the story, it gave you cases that related to it, and then it gave you the statutes that it broke or that it involved.

Young people were given written materials that clearly described their roles–what they needed to do and how it should be done. All of the "jobs" had clearly defined products to be completed before Model Assembly such as writing a bill, legal briefs, newspaper articles, and so on. This clarity of tasks and duties made it possible for young people to complete their work on time to be ready for Model Assembly.

Other support was given by youth veterans and by delegation advisors who provided practical advice and feedback when asked. All of this supported young people in going far beyond what they thought they were capable of. The invitation to participate does not stand alone; with it comes a variety of psycho-social and other supports. Together, these give young people safe adventure, travel into shaped wilderness parks, as it were, into the unknown with a guide, a first aid kit, a radio and a backup. Wilderness is only one spatial metaphor showing how the space of work was experienced and understood by participating youth.

By Creating a New Youth Geography

Involved young people learned much about how to do democracy because they were invited to work on what was meaningful to them. Another way to get at this is to understand this as space–both physical and activity. Young people in YIG talked about being able to take over the state capital building and appellate court rooms for their weekend.

You work for quite a few months on doing this and this is a big build-up and it's real for you, you're in the real court rooms, you have judges even though they're students but they're following the rules used by the big court, so it's a really cool experience because just thinking of where you are.

In PA they went to the field, the community, while in YSC the museum building became theirs: they had a security pass that allowed them building-wide access. Young people participated in new and different activities where they did what they might otherwise not have been allowed to try (Moss & Petrie, 2002); to them this was adult space. At times, young people were invited to enter this space, at other times their group made this decision.

> Just making the call, cause I didn't volunteer, and [my group] just said you should do this, and you're gonna do this now. That's probably one of the scariest things, because I didn't' want to do it at first, but then, when you get on the phone, it's just like any other phone call you make, just being like, yeah, well, how are you, um, is he there? And if he's not, you just hang up and try back later.

These new and different activities included making a phone call to an adult in their community, testifying at a school board meeting, researching case law at a university library, writing a letter to local and regional political officials, teaching science to community groups, meeting with community members, and launching a publicity campaign. Having the opportunity to enter exotic physical spaces and participate in democratic activity spaces that were both new and qualitatively different had real and positive consequences on their enjoyment, adventure and learning.

These multiple places were to them new, exciting and soon democratized spaces. In these places time too was democratized.

> I mean we've stayed on topic a lot of the times, but there's those weeks when nobody wants to do anything, and we sit there and we tell each other what we've been doing and why we don't want [to] do anything. So we're, we're kind of like counselors for each other, peer counselors, evaluators. . . . So, we get on task, and we get rolling and we get a lot of stuff done.

What may surprise those with a particular conception of youth as lazy and not able to plan is that these young people, when given the power to control their own time, got the work done.

In this program space, topic, and content were democratized.

> Participant: Right away, I thought we should go for more legalized fireworks, before, because that was our, we wanted to get more legalized, but then we had the guest speaker, and he just came in and then said that, and then we just changed it all to safety, and what we should do about them, and, probably stuff like that.

Interviewer: Alright, so the project, the what, of the project, right, what the project was, changed from legalizing more fireworks, to firework safety right?

Participant: Yeah.

Interviewer: How did that get changed?

Participant: Um, we, like after he came in, we just kind of stared at each other, and looked at the facts about like how many house fires, or like how many injuries last year, and we kind of just stared in awe about how much we didn't know about fireworks. And we're like, if we don't know that, how's the community gonna know either? Because, a lot of them didn't, and so, we go, well, oh, safety is always a big issue on everything, so that'd probably be a good one. It was.

Young people could choose what they would work on and as they learned about their topic, they often changed the focus of the work. By entering these spaces, young people were confronted with the "new" and the "strange," making them all the more ready to talk about what they were doing and how to get it done.

By Thinking About What We Are Doing

Young people talked a lot about reflecting on what they were doing. This reflection became ordinary because it was a part of how each project worked; it was more than an individual choice by staff, coaches or adults. So much of their experience in these initiatives, what they were asked to do, what they were allowed to do was new and this stimulated them to think about their work and their experience–what they were doing and how. These initiatives were not their taken-for-granted world (Way, 1998), neither "normal" nor "natural," and thus their work required greater concentration and effort than typical activities at school, home, religious place, and elsewhere in their neighborhoods. Asked to work in new spaces and to participate in new activities, they thought about what they were doing and what could happen if they were effective. Since they were not told how to accomplish their goals but, rather, guided and coached; their work strategy had to be figured out. They quickly learned that thinking about what they were going to do, what they were actually doing, and what they did (evaluation), improved their work and helped get it done well. This practical cognition was in the service of work and is a good example of instrumental thinking (e.g., Schon, 1983). Doing "real work," they do "real thinking." Why? To get the public work done and done well.

By Getting Public Work Done

Learning was not for learning's sake but was necessary to do the public work, their work as citizen. The public nature of the work provided feedback on their efforts, thus making it possible for them to evaluate and adapt what they were doing to context and moment. The public nature of their work, when joined to the reflective and evaluative way of working, enhanced the overall learning experience. Young people did not have to know what to do before beginning but figured out what to do over and over during the project. They knew when they had figured it out because real challenges, situations, and conditions changed. This ongoing negotiating with reality took different forms in each initiative, but it always met the definitional test of public work, "The expenditure of visible efforts by ordinary citizens whose collective labors produce things or create processes of lasting civic value" (Farr & Boyte, 1997, p. 42). They knew when they had succeeded because the work they did had a public ending in front of a public audience. Young people describe the many ways their work had larger public, civic meaning; it had public consequences–to a museum, a school or at the Model Assembly; it was for a public beyond them. While public work is never done, their event was time-limited, because the school term ended. Often their projects were incomplete when the time ended.

Reading Youth Civic Engagement Through Learning

These three civic education initiatives are powerful learning experiences which worked for young people. Why? Because young people were invited and supported in their work and in being unique individuals who could "make a difference." They were able to express their ideas publicly, be listened to, and to work in ways typically inaccessible to them because of their age. As legislators, scientists, and community servants, they gave to their communities–as persons, not as "youth." Age was marginalized and commitment and energy and enthusiasm were lived. They experienced being and doing citizen. Were these initiatives experiential education?

YOUTH CIVIC ENGAGEMENT AND EXPERIENTIAL EDUCATION

... Learning will happen more effectively if the learner is as involved as possible, using as many of his faculties as possible, in the learning; and that this involvement is maximized if the student has something that matters to him at stake. (Crosby, 1995, p. 5)

Taking this quote as a working definition of experiential education, all of the initiatives qualify. Young people's accounts of these initiatives provide concrete examples of how the philosophy and pedagogy of experiential education can be creatively applied and teach us, again, how we can support learning democratic practice.

From young people's accounts, learning emerged when they were supported, through invitation, reflection and action, to learn more about what they could do and to use their experience in these initiatives to make sense of both their past and who they were in new ways. At these moments, the initiatives provided a continuity of experience (Dewey, 1938) for participants. YSC and PA had the most success in bringing this about, in a large part because they worked on real issues and the roles young people played did not have to be returned when the experience ended. Young people in these two projects used these roles to name and envision themselves now and in their future. In YSC and PA, young people came away understanding themselves differently–they were not only students; they were also citizens, helpers, leaders, educators, researchers, and group facilitators.

In all three initiatives, adults and young people saw participants as having valuable previous experiences that they could draw upon. YSC and PA used these previous experiences explicitly–the projects groups worked on required young people to share what they believed, knew, and could do, even though individuals might not have recognized these before being in the group. In the three initiatives, young people came to see how they could use their past. By requiring youth to participate in meaningful actions that had public ramifications, young people learned what they could do now and what they might be able to do. In all initiatives, past experiences were either better understood (e.g., I didn't know I had this skill or knowledge) or transformed (e.g., I thought I couldn't but now realize that I can). All of this was done in ways that connected the past to possible future experience (e.g., I can do this again). While most experiential education in practice ends with reflection, what these initiatives illustrate is the power of going an additional step to applying what was learned (Kolb, 1984). This done, young people understood that what they learned was useful (Bruner, 1996).

They could easily apply what they learned because the initiatives were situated to make this possible. Their learning and its application took place in specific and, for the young people, real contexts. What made these real? Their work influenced others and vice versa (Dewey, 1938). Often these contexts were full of challenges and obstacles and the young people had to face and overcome these to get their work done; being successful at one's work required thinking through possibilities and also choosing to act on what they learned. These actions were immediately seen as useful or not. Deciding how to understand and respond to these challenges required analysis, reflection, exploration, and evaluation–learning.

Reflection is seen as basic to experiential education (Dewey, 1938; Kolb, 1984). From these initiatives we see how reflection can be scaffolded (Rogoff, 1990) in a variety of ways, both deliberate and non-deliberate (Moon, 2004). Deliberate reflection is what most experiential and informal educators are trained to do; it usually involves talking with participants before, during, and after an experience about the experience itself, their feelings of the experience, and what they might do differently next time (Jeffs & Smith, 1999). Non-deliberate reflection is what often happens due to surprising occurrences and/or encountering obstacles or challenges during an experience. It is non-deliberate because the experiential educator did not intentionally plan for it to happen. The space of activity (doing something in a new way) or place (entering a new location) invites participants to stop and think. Non-deliberate reflection is often the result of atypical work. Participants who have never done a type of work before take more time to think about what they are doing now and what they might do and how both relate to what they have already done. All is put into a time sequence, a biography of action and person.

Inviting young people into new and often strange activities and/or contexts did encourage them to reflect, although mostly in non-deliberate ways. This non-deliberate reflection was valuable for participants because it encouraged intentional actions. For them to complete their projects in the ways they were invited to do so was atypical, and this led many participants to proceed cautiously with each new task, pausing to see if what they just did worked, made sense, and moved the group's work forward. This was especially true when the group project met unexpected obstacles. These unexpected and surprising challenges caused participants to reflect. Often they were at a loss as to how they might maximize what they learned from meeting and overcoming these challenges; they needed help to make sense of it, to learn from it. While all initiatives excelled in providing scaffolds for non-deliberate reflection, allowing young people to engage in new and different activities, they had more difficulty sustaining and supporting deliberate reflection–naming important occurrences or observations and bringing them to the group for discussion. The exception was YSC where deliberate reflection occurred regularly in large part because skilled staff worked closely with small groups of young people over a long period.

Non-deliberate reflection flourished in part because these initiatives provided a non-mediated experience for young people (Moon, 2004). In each, young people talked about participating directly in the work. These projects were unusual in their invitation and support of young people's performance in challenging established roles. Young people encountered challenging and uncertain situations and had to figure it out (often in groups). These three initiatives were most powerful for young people when they did not have pre-determined endings. If the work was going to get done at all, the young people had to decide to do it and then to figure out ways of doing it well enough for it to be accepted as having been done "for real" in a context taken by them as real.

YOUTH CIVIC ENGAGEMENT AND SITUATED LEARNING

One useful way to make sense of these three initiatives is to look at them through the theory of situated learning (Lave & Wenger, 1991). While not true for all groups, many young people described these initiatives as more than taking part in a learning experience; they were also participating in a "community of practice" (Lave & Wenger, 1991). While there are many definitions of community of practice we use the term to refer to the joining of learning, practice, and identity (Reyes, 2006). Participants began these initiatives as novice participants, often in the company of more expert or master participants (Lave & Wenger, 1991). In both YIG and YSC, and for some groups in PA, novice participants did indeed work along side master participants (both adults and young people who had been involved in the work for a longer time). Through participating in the practice, they learned about it, the skills/knowledge necessary to complete it, and all the while exploring another possibility for who they are and could be–as young people and as adults (Zhu & Baylen, 2005). When young people were invited and supported in actual practice, they learned what it means to be a member and began to understand themselves as members. And this, young people said, made a huge difference. They belonged. This fit well with membership and belonging basic to democratic communities, to being and doing citizen.

These initiatives are similar in emphasizing learning through and in practice, guided by skilled others or self-instruction (Gieselman, Stark, & Farruggia, 2000). The focus of learning emerged from what they had to do. What they learned was how to get something they had to do done in a specific context (museum, school, or student-led government simulation). It was all contextual and situated. If formal training was involved, it was quickly put to use in practice. Participants were not trained or given information just for its own benefit or for general personal development, as is often the case in youth training programs. Instead, training directly related to what they needed and wanted to know and be able to do, so as to move along the group's project. Most often training took the form of simulation, as a type of practicing (Hung, Chee, Hedberg, & Seng, 2005). In all initiatives, participants often practiced what they had to do within the safe space of their group. They rehearsed their parts before they engaged in direct public performance. They often described this as planning and practicing what they had to do before doing it "live."

In these ways, these initiatives were philosophically and pedagogically experiential education (Dewey, 1938; Joplin, 1995; Kolb, 1984).

YOUTH CIVIC ENGAGEMENT OR CIVIC EDUCATION?

When are young people civically engaged? This question discloses the differences between civic education and youth civic engagement. Civic education is knowledge about our governmental system and its and our history, an understanding of the foundations of democracy and its underlying philosophy, a mastery of specific democratic skills (e.g., public speaking, critical thinking), and the taking on of particular values and beliefs (e.g., social responsibility, tolerance, compassion) (Butts, 1980; Patrick, 1996). Youth civic engagement challenges this conception of civic education; the key point is the emphasis put on learning and knowing-about versus on reflexive doing, primarily, being informed versus being engaged.

By describing the learning that takes place in these initiatives, we come to understand more clearly what engagement looks like. Clearly, young people who talked about these initiatives were engaged. This is true for all three of the initiatives, even the YSC, which did not have an explicit political focus, and YIG which ended too soon for the young participants. They were committed to these projects in ways unique and different from most of their other learning at home, school, or community; they took responsibility for themselves, each other, and their joint work. This engagement came out of the opportunity and the invitation to participate, coupled to their belief that they are worthy contributors with interest, commitment, energy, and the ability to "make a difference" in the public world on public issues. They were involved in a critical and what might be called emancipatory education opportunity (Freire, 1970; Hursh & Ross, 2000). These initiatives were important because within them, young people could become contributors to their community and school, and to their team members–each other. These initiatives work because youth are invited and supported in doing their work–collectively and individually.

Missing in all three initiatives is intentional reflection by adult and young people on how this work is citizen work. Clearly it is, yet most young people do not describe or name it as such. To them, they are "helping their communities" by being a senator, legislator, lawyer, scientist, or informal educator. They do not understand and make sense of their work in explicitly civic or political terms. Clearly this relates to the lack of intentional reflection on how and when their work is political or civic and on how and when they are democratic citizens. Possibly these are not illuminated because it is often assumed that because of their age they cannot be citizens. Or is it that few adults realize that this is indeed the work of democracy?

CITIZENSHIP AND EDUCATION

These initiatives illuminated important elements of good civic engagement teaching, what we call living citizenship. Those with the most powerful educational outcomes used experiential education (Gager, 1982; Kolb, 1984) within a situated learning frame (Lave & Wenger, 1991). They created supportive learning conditions (Dewey, 1938) in which young people had non-mediated experiences (Moon, 2004). When these conditions were met, young people learned what it meant to be a member, to do democratic civic practice, to be democratic citizen (Marker, 2000), and how to do and be this democratic citizen in everyday life.

All of the young people talked about how they learned to have a voice, work with others, and get stuff done. This is the stuff of citizenship and democratic civic practice (Boyte, 2004; Holden & Clough, 1998; Hursh & Ross, 2000). Missing and a source of why most youth do not talk about their work as citizen learning was deliberate reflection within the frames of democratic civic practice and living democratic citizen. They did not work to grasp how to take this democratic civic practice elsewhere in their life-worlds, school, home, and neighborhood. The possibility for such reflection existed but was not exploited.

What does this lack of reflection suggest? Clearly, these young people engaged in innovative civic work. They worked together to create lasting public outcomes. By any definition, they engaged in the work of democracy. How significant is it that they do not always describe what they have done as citizen work and who they are as citizens? This reveals more about the structures and institutions and the initiatives; we do not read this to mean that the initiatives failed. Rather, they succeeded in providing an invitation and system of support for young people to go beyond what we typically expect from them. Participants gained new skills, knowledge, and a sense of self. What often hinders further reflection and understanding of citizen is the limited conceptions of the adults and the failure to insure youth reflection through the lenses of and in the languages of politics, citizen, and youth civic engagement.

Missing too is a broader, more encompassing definition of citizen one that understands and defines parts of our everyday acts and activities as citizen work. Citizen is not something that sits apart from the everyday; rather it is found within everyday experiences and choices. Much of what young people did was not reflected on through the lens of citizen because it was often not understood by adults as being citizen work. Our definition of citizen is too weak, shallow, narrow and brittle.

Related is the image and understanding we have about young people. For many of us, citizen is equated with adulthood. This serves to keep childhood and youthhood a protected space where young people are not yet burdened with adult responsibilities, the issues and problems of civic life. Of course others simply believe young people to be incapable, uninterested, or unwilling to know and engage public issues. Our study surely contests the latter understanding and raises new questions for the former. Who gets to determine what is or is not appropriate responsibility for young people? It may be necessary to provide adequate protection for young people and not expect them to take on responsibilities often age-prescribed to adults. At the same time, how can we ensure that we are allowing them to use their capacities (Lansdown, 2006) for public benefit? These initiatives provide one answer to this question. A lot of effort has gone into building "developmentally appropriate" programs for young people; now we should focus on creating "capacity appropriate" programs as well. Young people told us these are the ones that contain the greatest possibility for their civic learning and civic engagement.

REFERENCES

Boyte, H. (2004). The necessity of politics. *Journal of Public Affairs, 7*(1), 75-85.

Bruner, J. (1996). *The culture of education.* Cambridge, MA: Harvard University Press.

Butts, R. F. (1980). The revival of civic learning: A rationale for citizenship education in American schools. Bloomington, IN: Phi Delta Kappa Educational Foundation.

Crosby, A. (1995). A critical look: The philosophical foundations of experiential education. In K. Warren, M. Sakofs, & J. S. Hunt (Eds.), *The Theory of Experiential education* (3rd ed., pp. 3-14). Dubuque, IA: Kendall/Hunt Publishing Company.

Dewey, J. (1938). Experience and education. New York: Collier Books.

Farr, J., & Boyte, H. (1997). The work of citizenship and the problem of service-learning. In R. Battistoni & W. Hudson (Eds.). *Experiencing citizenship: Concepts and models for service-learning in political science.* Washington DC: American Association for Higher Education.

Freire, P. (1970). *Pedagogy of the oppressed.* New York: The Continuum Publishing Company.

Gager, R. (1982). Experiential education: Strengthening the learning process. In D. Conrad & D. Hedin (Eds.), *Youth participation and experiential education.* New York: The Haworth Press.

Gieselman, J., Stark, N., & Farruggia, M. (2000). Implications of the situated learning model for teaching and learning nursing research. *The Journal of Continuing Education in Nursing, 31*(6), 263-268.

Holden, C., & Clough, N. (1998). *Children as citizens: Education for participation.* London: Jessica Kingsley Publishers.

Hung, D., Chee, T. S., Hedberg, J., & Seng, K. T. (2005). A framework for fostering a community of practice: Scaffolding learners through an evolving curriculum. *British Journal of Educational Technology, 36*(2), 159-176.

Hursh, D. W., & Ross, E. W. (Eds.) (2000). *Democratic social education: Social studies for social change.* New York: Falmer Press.

Jeffs, T., & Smith, M. (1999). *Informal education: Conversation, democracy and learning.* Derbyshire, UK: Education Now Publishing Co-operative Limited.

Joplin, L. (1995). On defining experiential education. In K. Warren, M. Sakofs, & J. Hunt, Jr. (Eds.). *The theory of experiential education.* Dubuque, IA: Kendall/Hunt Publishing Company.

Kolb, D. (1984). *Experiential learning: Experience as the source of learning and development.* Englewood Cliffs, NJ: Prentice-Hall, Inc.

Lansdown, G. (2006). *The evolving capacities of the child.* Florence, Italy: UNICEF Innocenti Research Centre.

Lave, J., & Wenger, E. (1991). *Situated learning: Legitimate peripheral participation.* Cambridge, U.K.: Cambridge University Press.

Marker, P. (2000). Not only by our words: Connecting the pedagogy of Paulo Freire with social studies curriculum. In D. W. Hursch & E. W. Ross (Eds.). *Democratic social education: Social studies for social change.* New York: Falmer Press.

Patrick, J. (1996). Principles of Democracy for the Education of Citizens. In J. Patrick & L. Pinhey (Eds.), *Resources on civic education for democracy: International perspectives* (pp. 5-17). Bloomington, ID: ERIC Clearinghouse for International Civic Education.

Reyes III, R. (2006). Cholo to 'me': From peripherality to practicing student success for a Chicano former gang member. *The Urban Review, 38*(2), 165-186.

Rogoff, B. (1990). *Apprenticeship in thinking: Cognitive development in social context.* New York: Oxford University Press.

Moss, P., & Petrie, R. (2002). *From children's services to children spaces.* London: Routledge/Falmer.

Schon, D. (1983). *The reflective practitioner: How professionals think in action.* New York: Basic Books.

Way, N. (1998). *Everyday courage: The lives and stories of urban teenagers.* New York: New York University Press.

Zhu, E., & Baylen, D. (2005). From learning community to community learning: Pedagogy, technology and interactivity. *Educational Medial International, 42*(3), 251-268.

The "Citizen" in Youth Civic Engagement

Is Youth Civic Engagement (YCE) really about citizenship? It depends on who you ask. The stated aim of each program in this study is, broadly speaking, to educate young people for democratic citizenship. Public Achievement's (PA) aim is to educate students to "become effective civic and political actors." Youth-in-Government's (YIG) stated aim is to "encourage life-long, responsible citizenship." The Youth Science Center's (YSC) aim is broader, "to promote healthy youth development" but also includes civic aims such as active participation in public and private institutions, responsibility, empowerment, and partnership. Yet there is a disjuncture between the official program descriptions and what young and older participants tell us these programs are about. In reading the youth and adult descriptions of these three programs, we are struck by the fact that participants rarely, if ever, use the language of politics or citizenship to describe their experiences. Instead, we heard a great deal about having a voice, doing something, working with others, and making a difference. What should we make of this? Is it a problem with the programs? Did they fail to meet their stated outcome of fostering democratic citizenship? Or did youth participate in activities that could be called *political* and come to new understandings of themselves which could be viewed in terms of *citizenship*, without using these words? Or does this point to something different, the fact that concepts used in political science to measure civic engagement are inadequate or incomplete?

This leads to an important query: given this absence, is it possible to "read" their statements in terms of politics, citizenship, democracy and the like? Here we answer yes! The ways in which young people talked about their experiences *can* be linked to concepts used in political science: participants were engaged in expressive activities, public action, cooperation, and attained a degree of political efficacy. Before turning to this reading, however, it is important to carefully consider the central concept of citizenship.

While each of these programs has the promotion of democratic citizenship as its mission, what do we mean when we use the term? What makes a particular form of citizenship democratic? More importantly, why does the meaning or definition of citizenship matter? In this chapter, we approach these questions from the perspective of political theory. Political theory, as an academic sub-discipline of political science and intellectual enterprise, is uniquely qualified to address these questions. It provides the critical and analytical tools to be more precise in how we talk about citizenship, to uncover taken for granted assumptions, to make implicit understandings explicit, and to offer normative frameworks to evaluate "good" citizenship. Though this discipline typically focuses on reading and re-reading canonical texts, we believe that it provides an important frame and the critical interpretive tools to read the three programs in question.

ACCOUNTS OF CITIZENSHIP

Citizenship is a contestable and, perhaps, even an essentially contested concept. While there are as many different visions of citizenship as there are political theories, there is some common ground regarding what a citizen is. A working standard definition of a citizen is a member or formally equal member of a political community who enjoys certain rights and privileges; is responsible for certain duties; has certain skills, capacities, virtues or attributes; and is engaged in certain public activities (e.g., Marshall, 1950). On one hand, this definition is helpfully broad, covering the expansive ground of citizenship. On the other hand, however, this breadth gives us little leverage to understand the actual practices of citizenship.

One alternative is to understand citizenship as a series of overlapping discourses that describe the relationship between an individual and a particular political community. Will Kymlicka and Wayne Norman (1995) draw the important distinction between three different discourses of citizenship: citizenship-as-legal-status, citizenship-as-desirable-activity, and citizenship-as-identity. Citizenship-as-legal-status refers to membership in a political community (p. 284). In both popular and academic discussions, citizenship-as-legal-status is directly linked to the nation-state. In this view, the nation-state confers legal status, is the source of rights and protections, and provides a collective identity. Recent debates over immigration, globalization, the war on terror, and ethnic minorities are central in discussions of citizenship-as-legal-status. However, as Kymlicka and Norman note, it is increasingly problematic to equate notions of a political community with the nation-state. The idea that the nation-state is the primary determinant of citizenship is being challenged from below (ethnic minorities) and above (international organizations, global capital).

Citizenship-as-desirable-activity refers to the idea that the "extent and quality of one's citizenship is a function of one's participation in that community" (p. 284). This discourse has clear normative dimensions, bringing into play the crucial question of what is a "good citizen." This question stimulates a divergent range of visions of the values, virtues, responsibilities, and dispositions of a "good citizen." These include but are not limited to critical (Bowles & Gintis, 1987), morally responsible (Colby, Ehlrich, Beaumont, & Stephens, 2003), tolerant (Gutmann, 1987), joining (Putnam, 2000), virtuous (Etzioni, 1992), knowledgeable (Hirsch, 1987, 1996), caring (Noddings, 1988), or justice-oriented (Westheimer & Kahne, 2004). Along with these normative ideals of citizenship, each also delineates a particular domain in which citizenship activities take place. Typically, ideal notions of citizenship are circumscribed within specific domains including formal political institutions or informal structures of civil society.

Citizenship-as-identity refers to how individuals view themselves and express their membership in a particular political community. While earlier conceptions of citizen identity were closely allied if not conflated with national identity or patriotism, recent theorists have challenged this "universalist" understanding of citizenship. Instead, they focus on the complex ways in which identity is constructed through difference. Iris Marion Young (1995) is probably the most important theorist of this perspective–variously called post-structural, cultural pluralist, or multi-cultural. Young presents a convincing argument how conceptions of universal citizenship have been used to systematically exclude certain social groups. Even though oppressed groups have used the ideal of equal citizenship in their hard efforts to be included as citizens, the strict adherence to principle of equal treatment tends to perpetuate oppressions of disadvantage (p. 250). She calls for a new idea of differentiated citizenship–that oppressed social groups should be able to organize themselves and be ensured representation in political processes. What is more important, for our purposes, is that new post-structural and multi-cultural perspectives reveal that identity is always constituted in relation to difference, both internally and externally. It also highlights the social nature in the construction of citizenship–we define ourselves by what we are not. This argument breaks apart the notion that human beings are unitary actors, in favor of a notion of possessing multiple selves, one of which could be as citizen.

RESEARCH ON CIVIC ENGAGEMENT

Kymlicka and Norman's account of the three discourses of citizenship is reflected in much of the empirical research on youth civic engagement. In recent years there has been an explosion of research that seeks to measure young people's political and civic attitudes, knowledge, skills, and dispositions (Billig, 2000; Delli Carpini & Keeter, 1996; Eyler & Giles, 1999; Keeter, Zukin, Andolina & Jenkins, 2002; Neimi & Junn, 1998; Mann & Patrick, 2000; Torney-Purta, 2002). This scholarship is typically conducted through large studies that seek to measure political knowledge, attitudes, skills, or to measure changes that result from particular "interventions." To take one example, Keeter, Zukin, Andoline, and Jenkins (2002) provided an important framework for measuring the "civic and political health" of American youth. Through survey research, this team examined the extent in which people report political or civic behaviors. They divided their research into civic indicators (community problem solving, volunteering, membership in a group or association, raising money for charity, participating in walks), electoral indicators (voting, persuading others, displaying buttons or signs, campaign contributions, or working for political campaigns), and expressive indicators (contacting officials, contacting the media, protesting, on-line or written petitions, boycotting, or canvassing). Except for, perhaps, on measures of community problem solving, Keeter and associates may *not* find that many participants in PA, YIG, and YSC are civically engaged! YIG participants would probably score well on studies that seek to measure political content (knowledge of how democratic institutions work). Outcomes from programs like PA and YSC where youth co-create the projects, activities, and processes often do not easily map onto standardized studies.

We believe that these standard approaches to "measuring" citizenship are useful for understanding the broader landscape about youth. We disagree with the conclusions of scholars such as Stephen E. Bennett (1997) that young people are apathetic and hate politics (p. 47). While Bennett is intending to provoke action, we believe such conclusions may contribute to the current moral panic about youth. More importantly, we think that these research methods suffer from being too narrow and for failing to take into account the everyday contexts in which these activities take place. By narrow, we mean that researchers define *in advance* what activities, behaviors, and attitudes count as civic engagement. As noted in the introduction, this narrowing has the consequence of not "seeing" certain forms of activity or ways of being as political. The result is that many studies find that young people are not politically and civ-ically engaged (insofar as those terms are defined by researchers) and also conclude that youth are apathetic. In addition, large sample studies, by design, control for context. They also seek to measure disembodied indicators of knowledge, attitudes, and skills. Changes in these indicators are measured in relation to scales set by researchers, not in relation to the lived experiences of young people.

READING YOUTH CIVIC ENGAGEMENT (YCE) THROUGH THE LENS OF CITIZENSHIP

Recall that standard discourses of citizenship focus on *what* citizens *are* (legal status), what they *should do* (desirable activity), and *how* they *identify* as citizens (collective identity). From our reading of the lived experiences of young people in these three initiatives, we came to see that these standard discourses miss something very important–they miss the embedded, embodied, and dialectical relationship between *doing*, *being* and *becoming* citizen in a specific life-world. Thus we offer *lived citizen* as a critical expansion and bridging dimension to current discourse of citizenship. We are not the first to call for an expanded definition of citizenship. In an 1897 address to educators, John Dewey (1972) declared,

> To isolate the formal relationship of citizenship from the whole system of relations with which it is actually interwoven; to suppose that there is any one particular study or mode of treatment that can make a child a good citizen; to suppose, in other words, that a good citizen is anything more than a thoroughly efficient and serviceable member of society, one with all his powers of body and mind under control, is a cramped superstition which is hoped may soon disappear from educational discussion. (p. 59)

While Dewey's hope that this "cramped superstition" would disappear is unfulfilled, it is worth revisiting his work, among others, to read these initiatives. In the rest of the chapter we draw on Dewey as well as Hannah Arendt to offer a reading of these three initiatives.

The Domain of Citizenship: The Public Realm

An important common theme to all three initiatives was the domain of activities–where they happened and how they defined their work. As noted in chapter 5, we paid careful attention to the context, both the young peoples' everyday lives and the context of the respective programs. First and foremost, participants from every program noted that "this was different than school" or "something new." In these programs young people worked with others, often with people they never met before. This resonates with Hannah Arendt's (1958) understanding of the public realm. She characterizes the public realm as the space of politics where people encounter the plurality of other humans and take action and build power through collective endeavors. Rather than locating "the political" solely within political institutions or prescribed activities such as voting, Arendt holds that politics takes place wherever people act in concert. Here we can see an important shift in how we understand citizenship and civic engagement. In chapter 7 we discussed how each program embodied an invitation for learning. This invitation can also be viewed in terms of an invitation to joint endeavor, an invitation that can take place in any setting–at work, in school, in extra-curricular programs, even in families.

It is through working with others in the public realm that young people experienced themselves being able to express themselves, to have a voice, to give their input, and to have (collective) control over the PA group, YSC exhibit, or how the YIG model assembly turned out. This quote is typical:

> In PA . . . you can actually voice your opinion and do basically what you want to do. But in other things, it's other people above you saying that you can do this or you can do that, but you still have your right to voice your opinion, but then there's a higher authority saying you can't do this or you can't do that. But basically in PA, let it be your thing, and it was your peers that said they didn't want to do this or they didn't want to do that.

YSC participants commented on the openness of their experiences, how you can suggest and then do anything. This expectation was based on the ethos and approach of all initiatives–participants all understood that they had significant control as to how to carry out their work. Each program was intentionally structured to allow this, to varying degrees.

Beyond this programmatic design for student input and expression, our interviews revealed three additional dimensions that contributed to opening a public realm for young people–control over the course of their activities, being taken seriously (listened to), and being able to show the world that they can "make a difference." Students' lived experiences of voice and control are contrasted with the constraint they feel in the rest of their lives in school. It may be that the idea that "everyone can contribute" alters the disciplinary effects of knowledge in school (typically experienced in terms of being right or wrong). Thus, new spaces for expression are opened when the typical role of student was disrupted.

Instead of being instructed by a teacher, young people collaborated with adult coaches, co-workers, or experienced youth participants.

Young people experienced themselves as being listened to and taken seriously by other young people and adults. They felt that their ideas would influence how their projects, exhibits, or assembly decisions would turn out. This quote is typical: "Cause this made me feel like, you know, my voice can be heard and other people could go along with my opinion. And I could affect them and, you know, have them want to do something too." Our interviews revealed the often forgotten counterpart to political expression: listening. One young person told us that he rarely feels listened to in his everyday life, "but in Public Achievement, they was like, they were listening. They understand." The lived experience of being listened to is central not only to being taken seriously but reaching a sense of mutual understanding among young people and adults.

Finally, young people told us that it was important to show the world that young people can do "important things." This starts with the seemingly mundane trope of young people in PA and YSC saying how "It was important to do things" or "What I liked is we got things done." But when we listen further, it is through getting things done that age/grade expectations were altered for these students. Consider the response that "I did learn that, like, just because we are younger and not adults yet, we can still make a difference in the world." Young people often drew the attention to how they think adults and the broader world perceive them (as not caring about their school/community or not being serious public actors). This underscores the public dimension to agency. Not only are youth doing things in public, they are showing the public that youth *can* do things. This sentiment was more pronounced at inner-city schools where this sentiment extends beyond "youth as youth" to include urban youth and/or youth of color. These students talked about PA as a chance to show adults and the broader world that not all students at their school are "thugs."

Returning to Arendt (1958), she argues that it is only in the public realm that people can "appear" before one another in a way that both affirms their individuality and the common world they share (pp. 57-58). This opening, this space of expression, of working with others, of being listened to, of collective control all contribute to young people coming to see themselves in a new way, to experience themselves as efficacious, to have this new sense be witnessed by the rest of the group and hopefully come to see themselves in a new way as citizens. In a very important way Arendt is reconfiguring typical discourses of citizen identity. Rather than being defined as a member of a nation state or in terms of identities of difference, Arendt looks at citizen identity in terms of the modes of being in the world defined by speech and action. As we will discuss in chapter 10, youth are often "seen" and thereby defined in developmental terms. Through speech and action, young people "insert" themselves into the public realm. This insertion carries both the risk and reward of disclosure–they will show the world "who" they are. This takes courage! Arendt notes that an individual does not act in public with the intention of "showing" the world who they are; rather one's uniqueness is disclosed through taking action. How does this work? For Arendt, the first element of disclosure is that the outcome of public actions can never fully be known. Things may turn out differently than we expect! In this sense we may disclose to the world our competence or incompetence (p. 192). The second element is that our uniqueness needs to be seen, witnessed and discussed by others. Rather than defining ourselves via difference, our distinctness is revealed through working with others. Our interviews revealed that young people have demonstrated forms of competence that break age-grade expectations. They understand this in the sense that others (other group members, adults, teachers) see them differently. This presence of others is a critical dimension in the relationship between doing, becoming, and being lived citizen.

The Activities of Citizenship: Interactions with the World

A second important theme was that through civic engagement young people interacted in and with the world in new ways. Our use of interaction relies heavily on the philosopher John Dewey. Experience, defined as the interaction between an individual and their natural and social environments, is a central concept in Dewey's broader philosophical work. Dewey is helpful here because he takes seriously the everyday experience as a source of both learning and democratic engagement. Dewey is considered a seminal figure in experiential education literature and provided an early account of how learning occurs. He conceives of learning in terms of a cycle of encountering problematic situations, diagnosing, constructing hypotheses about how to address the problem, taking action to test one's hypotheses, and reflecting on what happened. Learning, for Dewey, comes from understanding the significance or meaning of our interactions with the environment. In its most basic sense, meaning comes from understanding the connections between actions and consequences.

For young people in PA and YSC, the learning that came from mundane tasks such as contacting museum officials or preparing legislative briefs was crucial. In Deweyan terms, the "trying" of talking to the museum official was followed by the "undergoing" of being listened to and taking seriously by adults. This experience resulted in furthering their group's work as well changing how they saw themselves. When asked what they can do now that they could not do before, students would launch into a list of what could be labeled civic skills. While students tended not to describe their work in terms of political terms, they did have an understanding of how learning skills opened a horizon of possibility where they saw that they could "do things" and "make a difference" in the world. Even though they did not name "making a difference" in political terms, there are clear political dimensions to this idea.

When framed in the terms of political theory, the outcome of these interactions are clearly examples of political agency. Many students already experienced themselves as agents within the group, being able to express themselves and seeing how their ideas influenced the group's broader work. This theme of interaction draws a qualitative difference between PA and YSC from the simulated experiences of YIG. Though each program was experienced as "real" and "meaningful" for participants, PA and YSC involved interaction with the "public." Even though we are interacting "with the world" all the time, PA and YSC groups interacted with individuals and institutions beyond the confines of their groups. We have learned that there are several distinct dimensions that contribute to young peoples' lived experiences of political agency.

First, young people in PA and YSC told us many stories about the challenges of doing seemingly mundane tasks–like making a phone call. Many younger students (but a surprising number in high school, as well) talked about how nervous they were making a phone call. Some students had scripts and practiced before their conversations, though many did not. The outcomes of the initial phone calls were mixed. Some went really well and students found that adults responded positively. Others were more difficult, with students not knowing what to say or adults not taking them seriously. Students would reflect with the coach, other team members, or supervisor on their difficulties and try again. There were numerous students who talked about how important it was for them to learn how to make phone calls. We suggest that it is not the phone call itself that is difficult–young people make phone calls all the time–but interacting with adults outside of their typical social roles.

Second, young people saw that their individual and collective actions had consequences for the project and their group. Here we see the importance in Dewey's method of cooperative inquiry–it is through collectively taking action, testing hypotheses, reflecting on consequences, and devising new forms of action that learning occurs. For PA, actions like meetings with principals produced immediate feedback–groups could either proceed with their planned action or they could not. When principals or site personnel did not approve projects, students and coaches would often evaluate and come up with a different plan of action. A fifth grader in PA learned that "Well, if you want something in this school, you shouldn't just go up to the principal and say, 'I want this.' You should get the other people that want the same thing as you and [have them] sign a letter [showing their support]." Students thus saw the real consequences of *not* getting work done. Many reported learning a new sense of accountability–not to teachers, parents or grades–but to their group's progress and to each other.

Third, students experienced agency through the difficult process of carrying out complex projects with multiple steps. A major challenge that all PA and YSC teams encountered was learning about and doing all the intermediate steps and logistical work needed before they could do their projects. A common experience for group members was learning that things take longer than expected and involved many more steps than expected. The bureaucratic systems of schools and museums are not easy to negotiate; this difficulty is magnified when individual students or groups did not complete assigned tasks. But, as Dewey (1983) notes, an important dimension of learning comes from encountering resistance from the world or, as he says, "run up against the actual world of hard conditions" (p. 26) This resistance often came from dealing with individuals, organizations, or bureaucratic systems. One important contrast between the initiatives is that in PA, students often commented they had problems with principals, teachers, or vendors who did not take the students and/or their issue seriously. In YSC, youth were nearly universal in feeling that museum staff took them seriously. Another important theme was being forced to change goals, strategies, projects, and even focal issue topics mid-course. In the course of carrying out projects, planning and evaluation became important components of agency. There were stops and starts, obstacles and wrong turns but, through trying things out, revising, and trying them again students learned that they could (or what they needed to do to) complete their projects. In fact, many were surprised that they accomplished what they did.

DOING, BECOMING, AND BEING CITIZEN

The final and most important theme is an examination of how these programs help young people become and be active citizens. This means going beyond "doing citizen" (participating in programs) to "being citizen." We entitled the book "being while becoming" to denote the complex an always inter-related process of becoming and being in the formation of the civic self. In our interviews, we tried to "touch" this phenomenon by asking about the ways young people integrated what they learned through these programs and activities into their everyday lives. For us, this represents the real test of these programs and of YCE in general.

The empirical literature on youth civic engagement has not been able to definitively answer this question (Hepburn, 2000). While there is data on the mastery of civic knowledge, attitudes and skills, there is little on whether young people, in the words of the literature, take on "civic dispositions." The theoretical literature has tended to examine this question through the concept of identity. This literature has proven more robust in thinking through the construction of citizenship through difference but does not readily translate to the everyday lived experiences of young people.

In the introductory chapter we offered the term "lived citizen" as a way to think beyond standard discourses of citizenship and standard frameworks for viewing youth towards conceiving citizenship in terms of vocation. Here we look to Dewey's writing on vocation to help us think through the relationship between doing, becoming and being active citizen. This section is admittedly tentative. Our interviews disclosed the rich and textured learning experiences of youth participants in PA, YIG, and YSC but did not (and possibly could not) reveal much movement from learning through doing to a sense of becoming/being lived citizen. Yet it is important to engage in this normative task of thinking through the ways in which citizenship can become lived.

Dewey reconstructed the concept of vocation during debates over industrial or trade training in the 1910s and 1920s. He was a vociferous critic of "trade training" and called for a re-thinking of the term vocation in ways that restored its earlier meanings. Dewey's concept of vocation draws together his notions of interests and habits. For Dewey, interests signify the transactive connections between an individual and the world. In making this claim, Dewey draws on the Latin understanding of interest as *inter esse* meaning "in between." This stands in contrast to ordinary usage where self-interest is understood as a kind of selfish attachment to an object and altruism is understood when a person acts without interest, or unselfishly. Dewey says that both self-interest and altruism are based on a false assumption: that the "self" is fixed and forged before acting with the world. Moreover, Dewey (1985) believes that the self is always in "continuous formation through choice of action" (p. 361). This notion of a self-always-on-process reconfigures how we conceive of interests. In this sense, interests are a *means*; they account for *how* we become interested in particular ends.

While interests are clearly an important part to civic engagement, they are not enough. Without habits to structure and sustain our interests, Dewey argues that we would simply drift from one interest to another. Our habits structure our particular experiences; a vocation or calling orders and structure the "immense diversity" of experiences in a *particular* direction. Habits are also, for Dewey, expressions of learning and growth (p. 49). As such, they are crucial for understanding and recon-structing what it means to learn, in general, and to learn active citizenship, in particular. Our interests in this sense are buttressed by habits–they provide the ready-to-hand means to interpret and respond to our social situations.

Taken together, interests and habits coalesce into a rich concept of vocation. Dewey uses the vocational notion of a "calling" as a way of organizing habits in a particular direction. He elaborates, "A calling is an organizing principle for information and ideas; for knowledge and intellectual growth. It provides an axis which runs through an immense diversity of detail; it causes different experiences, facts, items of infor-mation to fall into order with one another" (p. 319). One of Dewey's main innovations to educational debates in the beginning of the twentieth century was to define vocation as plural: we have many different vocations that correspond to the many different environments in which we live (e.g., a person may define themselves in terms of being a teacher, husband, parent, photographer, etc.).

For Dewey, the concept of vocation refers to the particular constellation of interests and habits that are an integral part of who we are. To put it differently, we could not be ourselves if we were not following our calling. When we are living our vocation, or following our calling, we both lose and find ourselves in that particular object or activity. "In fact," Dewey continues, "self and interest are two names for the same fact; the kind and amount of interest actively taken in a thing reveals and measures the quality of selfhood which exists (p. 362). This continuous development of "interesting" experiences, of "losing and finding oneself" in a particular activity, coalesces into a sense of vocation. Vocation, in this sense, refers to the "the active moving *identity* of the self with a certain object" (p. 362).

We believe that thinking in terms of democratic habits and civic vocations opens up new ways of thinking about youth civic engagement. We advance the hypothesis that persons living citizenship will be able to "hear the call" of the political world, to read certain situations in public and political terms, and to be able to respond in public and political ways. We can easily think of times when we were so engrossed that we lost track of time yet, at the same time, we were never more ourselves by doing this particular activity. The hope is that citizenship can be one (of many) vocations. Perhaps most importantly, Dewey's use of habits, interest, and vocation opens up space and movement to understand the relation to what we do as citizens and the process of becoming/being a living citizen. As noted in the introductory chapter, we believe that there are deeper sources to understand this concept of vocation. While Dewey offers the beginning grounds to think through the process of becoming an active citizen, in next chapter we explore the concept of vocation in more detail.

CONCLUSIONS

In our readings of these three initiatives through the lens of political theory, we have highlighted how Dewey and Arendt provide an alternative framework for citizenship and politics. Arendt's understanding of the public realm as a space where people come together in work and deed opens up alternate and surprising domains for citizenship. However, as Arendt notes, the public realm is increasingly being squeezed out by social and commercial concerns. Therefore, public realms need to be created. One important role of each initiative is to embody this invitation, to provide this space where people can come together. These spaces, as we have seen, are characterized by varying degrees of freedom for youth to pursue their own agendas. Our discussion of Dewey highlighted the importance of interaction in these public spaces, both within groups or teams and with the "real" world. Dewey's account of interaction reveals how the experiences in these initiatives are a source for learning and civic growth. This reading of Arendt and Dewey provides a more grounded, embodied, and fluid understanding of the relationship between *doing* citizen activities (PA, YIG, and YSC), *becoming* citizen (learning through interaction), and *being* citizen.

REFERENCES

Arendt, H. (1958). *The human condition.* Chicago: University of Chicago Press.

Bennett, S. (1997). Why young Americans hate politics, and what we should do about it. *PS: Political Science and Politics, 30*(1), 47-52.

Billig, S. (2000). Research on K-12 school-based service-learning: The evidence builds. *Phi Delta Kappan, 81,* 658-664.

Bowles, S., & Herbert, G. (1976). *Schooling in capitalist America: Educational reform and the contradictions of economic life.* New York: Basic Books.

Colby, A., Ehrlich, T., Beaumont, E., & Stephens, J. (2003). *Educating citizens:Preparing America's undergraduates for lives of moral and civic responsibility.* San Francisco, CA: Jossey-Bass.

Delli Carpini, M. X., & Keeter, S. (1996). *What Americans know about politics and why it matters.* New Haven, CT: Yale University Press.

Dewey, J. (1972). *The early works, 1882-1898* (Volumes 1-5). Jo Ann Boydston, ed. Carbondale, IL: Southern Illinois University Press.

Dewey, J. (1983). *The middle works, 1899-1924* (Volume 1: 1899-1901). Jo Ann Boydston, ed. Carbondale, IL: Southern Illinois University Press.

Etzioni, A. (1992). *The spirit of community: Rights, responsibilities, and the communitarian agenda.* New York: Crown Publishers.

Eyler, J., & D. Giles. (1999). *Where's the learning in service-learning?* San Francisco: Jossey-Bass.

Gutmann, A. (1987). *Democratic education.* Princeton, NJ: Princeton University Press.

Hepburn, M. (2000). Service learning and civic education in the schools: What does recent research tell us? In S. Mann & J. Patrick (Eds.), *Education for civic engagement in Democracy.* Bloomington, IN: ERIC.

Hirsch, E. D. (1987). *Cultural literacy: What every American needs to know.* New York: Vintage Books.

Hirsch, E. D. (1996). *The schools we need: And why we don't have them.* New York: Random House.

Keeter, S., Zufkin, C., Andolina, M., & Jenkins, K. (2002). *The civic and political health of a nation: A generational portrait.* New York: Pew Charitable Trusts.

Kymlicka, W., & Norman W. (1995). Return of the citizen: A survey of recent work on citizenship theory. *Ethics, 104,* 352-381.

Mann, S., & Patrick, J. (2000). *Education for civic engagement in democracy: Service learning and other promising practices.* Bloomington, IN: Educational Resources Information Center.

Marshall, T. H. (1950). *Citizenship and social class.* Cambridge: Cambridge University Press.

Neimi, R., & Junn, J. (1998). *Civic education: What makes students learn.* London: Yale University Press.

Noddings, N. (1984). *Caring: A feminine approach to ethics and moral education.* Berkeley and Los Angeleos: University of California Press.

Putnam, R. (1995). Tuning in, tuning out: The strange disappearance of social capital in Aamerica. *PS: Political Science & Politics, 28,* 664-684.

Torney-Purta, J. (2002). The school's role in developing civic engagement: A study of adolescents in twenty-eight countries. *Applied Developmental Science, 6*(4), 203–212.

Westheimer, J., & Kahne, J. (2004). "Educating the "good" citizen: Political choices and pedagogical goals. *PS: Political Science and Politics, 37*, 241-247. Accessed on May 3, 2005, http://www.apsanet.org

Young, I. M. (1995). Polity and group difference: A critique of the ideal of universal citizenship. In R. Beiner (Ed.), *Theorizing Citizenship*. Albany, NY: State University of New York Press.

"I Want to Make a Difference"

In this chapter, we work at understanding this most common answer young people gave to the question of why they took on and treated seriously the role of "public worker" (Boyte & Farr, 1997) in their school's Public Achievement (PA) initiative. At first glance, this topic is so commonsensical that it suggests at most a five page essay. But this turns out to be wrong, as we pursue these particular young persons' account of this intentional action.

The major orienting questions are:

- What are young people saying when they give this answer?
- How can we make sense of what they are saying?

When individual young people answer the question, "Why did you get involved and stay involved in PA?" most say it is because or "in order to" make a difference on a particular social issue or problem, typically in their neighborhood or community, often in the school and, at times, in the larger world (Cresswell, 2004). Examples of these issues and problems are shown in Table 9.

Let's look closely at this response. "I want (to)" says: I chose to (not I need to or I must), an existential self-commitment and an existential statement of one's freedom, a free crafting of one's time/space and self. I want to may also mean *I should* and along with "should" comes because and/or in order to–situated, everyday answers to the question why or reasons for doing what I did. In academic terms these responses are accounts (Mills, 1963; Tilly, 2006), I want to asserts but leaves unsaid the source of this "It's why?" in personal meaning, experience, motive, thought and/or feeling.

To "I want" add "to make," that is, to do, to build and, as is typical in our data, to fix, to repair (Spelman, 2002): construction, action, change, power, the notion of efficacy, and the like. This says also, "I can make," "I am able to make;" it serves to make *make* a node of knowledge/power/action/meaning.

Make what? A difference, youth say, make someplace, some condition or some thing better. Often this means less bad and it also means more good: less crime, less dumping of trash; more street safety, with cleaner and better lighted streets. Young people want to make a difference in how their worlds look and work and to make a difference for others as well as

TABLE 9. Issue, Concern, Problem

Issue	Concern	Problem
Clean School	Littering	Entrance is full of fast food containers
Health	Dead animals	Dead cats left on my street
Health	Fast food	No healthy food in school cafeteria
Well-being of others	Abuse	Don't know enough about abuse of teenagers

for themselves and their friends, for example, by creating safe spaces for themselves and their friends. These others are often called the community and to young people this can mean a geographic place and/or a specific ethnic-racial, language, or life-style group, e.g., African-Americans, poor folks, children, or skateboarders.

The phrase, "I want to make a difference" means to some that they want to be known as the person who made the space better; to some it means that they want others to gain from their work. Some youth see themselves acting in ways that they hope other youth will emulate, i.e., do positive things for our community and turn things around. Much of this is heard in their phrases, "I do this because" and "I do it in order to," two themes in situational accounts (Lyman & Scott, 1989). Both themes are found in youth responses to the question, "Why do you do this?"

Why indeed do young people get involved and work at making a difference in school, neighborhood, and community? Because and in-order-to are the two main forms of account they offer, as shown. To some these are public answers that do not fully account for private motives and reasons. Looking at these, young people tell about wanting things to be better for themselves and for those who will come after them, showing a grasp of future continuity and legacy too often unsuspected as theirs; wanting something that happened to them not to happen to others and as a way of dealing with ugly things in their own biographies and everyday lives.

Another type of reason given is that such work is fun, interesting, "not school" (which is "boring" and mostly "irrelevant"). Related too is that they learn relevant and important skills, stuff that will help in life such as analyzing a real problem, planning and organizing with others, public speaking, and contacting (adult) public officials. A part of this is having and using power to "get things done" and to "make things happen," which is basic to making a positive difference in the worlds of school and street.

Many young people see their work and their wish to make a difference as a type of responsibility–what goes along with, for some, being a citizen, while for others what it means to be a religious person. Of course, some young people merge the two: civic duty and religious obligations are stated as:

- "I do it in order to make things better."
- "I do it because this is what a religious person (a good Christian) should do."

This last account, as expected, was found to be most common, real and powerful among (private) Catholic school students and African-Americans in private and public schools. It was these young people who were most experienced in group decision-making and social action likely, we suspect, because of their involvement in community religious youth activities.

Young people across the four U.S. states (Kansas, Minnesota, Missouri, Wisconsin) and also in Northern Ireland (along with other youth from violent and post-violent societies in Europe and Africa) all gave at minimum this same reason: I want to make a difference. We heard this so often we came to paradoxically fully believe it as spoken by (almost) every young person and also to fully doubt that it was a real, true, authentic response. Was this simply a common socially normative response learned and practiced in school and elsewhere by young people, a way to close the question and the encounter with a probing adult? Was it that alone? Or was it a true, real, and authentic statement of the self? Was it public idiom and private meaning, the sociopolitical, the philosophical, the religious and the psychological? Bullshit or truth or both? Was it a true way of naming oneself and not a way to get rid of me, to "cool me out" or to con oneself?

The social sciences offer one approach to making sense of their answer.

MAKING SENSE

Their response is so reasonable, typical, American, and seemingly cross-national that it is rarely reflected upon by adults, except when it is heard as bullshit, what you are supposed to say, a con. These interpretations come into play when the young person does not seem to be the type who would really believe that, is known as a young person whose demeanor and/or behavior does not fit with this motive, is someone who in the moment of the question and answer is experienced (and read) as putting us on, as inauthentic, as gaming. That is, we interpret and accept or reject this response based in part on knowing the particular youth or judging him or her based on our take on youth like her or him. That is, the answer or response is taken as an account and this we assess based on how we read him or her. We accept the reason or not; we or may not this as the true or real motive.

There is a social science of such situated and unsituated accounts, disclaimers, reasons and explanations in the contexts of understanding and of scientific explanations (Mills, 1940; Tilly, 2006). In a deep sense this is about truth, meaning, interpretation, cause, and a related set of scholarly and practical issues, far too many and seemingly too far away from our direct concerns of how to hear and make sense of the phrase, "I want to make a difference." But this literature can be used to approach their response.

And for us it proved useful but unsatisfying. There seemed to be more here than those analytic frames and categories could get at. There is more here than cause or motive, we sense. A far older and richer approach was to take the question for a walk inside a more holistic conception of person: vocation.

Vocation

Vocation is a venerable notion in Western, Northern thought, the belief that one can be called to live life in particular ways best suited to oneself. Used to understand work as a social station, a social role in current terms, vocation joined person to world through God: one was called to a social position–farmer, tradesman, religious person and, after discerning his call as true, lived as farmer, or better, became farmer–took on the occupation, the place where he lived, his way of being farmer, his way of being himself–his very doing and being–the praxis that is him; he was farmer, through and through. Martin Luther revised vocation in the 1500s and the notion was applied generously to women too and mother, wife, craftsperson also became social stations, valid, spiritually imbued, and socioreligously important. Max Weber used vocation to discuss politics (Gerth & Mills, 1958), and the authors of *Habits of the Heart* (Bellah, 1986), a recent, now classic exploration of civic engagement, also refer to vocation. It is a notion at home in analyzing and understanding and explaining citizen work philosophically, sociologically, psychologically, and in everyday practical terms.

Vocation is historico-spatial–it works in time and place inviting, indeed compelling, those who discern a true call to take up work here and now in occupational and social roles available in the community, in everyday life. Vocation in its spiritual meaning-world and in secular usage is about doing work one must take on in one's everyday world. One must become who one must in the here and now–do the work and become the person. This is neither destiny nor fate but a living response to a higher call and claim: this is who one must work at becoming, doing, and being–a praxis of self.

How can the young person's phrase, "I want to make a difference" be read through vocation? What does such a reading tell about the phrase as such, about citizenship, and about civic duty? Here vocation is in conversation with citizen. Reciprocally, what does the phrase and our data teach about vocation and the vocational?

THE PHRASE

To begin with a rephrasing: I am called to make a difference in my school, i.e., to make things better; that is, to make the streets safe for walking and playing. Or I see as my purpose or my mission-in-life to make things better for my community. These rephrasings bring the most common reason for civic action directly into the language-world of vocation. Seen here is a shift from personal motive in a psychological and/or moral sense to the commitment of self, of the whole person. Reworded as "This is what I must do," the phrase now picks up the self's experience of a compelling commitment to act in a certain way. Vocation is a way, a path, a shape of the self, a response. To what? A call. And a self-life shaped by and through one's response to a call or to the world's address. It is reasonable and effective to use vocation as a language-world for understanding young people's explanations for their civic engagement and their given reasons for their commitment. Theirs is a vocational commitment in the language-world of the vocation of citizen.

In classic terms, vocation was tied to stations of life, specifically to social roles, among these gender, race, and age. Indeed, vocation can be joined to age in a radical interrogation of the concepts youth, young person, and young people. In our society, all children, adolescents, and youth study civics and citizenship, with few actually living civic roles in their everyday lives. Those with such lived-experience are exposed to and may come to master the skills, beliefs, and practice-wisdom of citizen-work, of public work (Boyte & Skelton, 1997). Because there is no national requirement that young people be involved, participate, or engage in civic affairs in school, neighborhood, or elsewhere in their life-worlds, these skills, beliefs and wisdom are not constitutive elements of the social role youth nor are they in the knowledge and skill repertoire of most young people. But these could be, and it is to this end that initiatives such as PA work with schools and their students (young people). These could be a general and widespread *age-specific* social station called youth civic activist, as there is now among subgroups in the U.S. and internationally.

Classically, vocation joined person to God on one side and to the world on the other. This was seen among African-American youth who were active in their religious congregations, where they were given real and meaningful responsibilities for church structure and program, and it was also found among youth involved in organized youth programs in their religious communities. Broadening vocation from a call to include the address of the world opens the possibility that any young person can be called upon or confronted or addressed by what happens in near to far worlds, in at-hand and more distant life-worlds. Does she or he notice the world calling? How does she or he do this? What sense does she or he make of the invitation? How does she or he figure out what she or he wants to or has to do in response? What does she or he do? All of this, and more, may go into *discerning* whether or not the individual experiences a claim made on her by world-facts, world-ills, world-hurt: violence, injustice, garbage on the streets, drug dealing, and the like–the stuff, the fact, one wants to change for the better as a way of making a difference. In this view, one's lives are in constant, renewable dialogue with the world (and, for some, also with God) and it is in and through these ongoing conversations that one becomes, is, and renews oneself as the person one is: *who* we are is *how* we act in response to the address of the world. Lived-vocation is one's identity, one's self; it is one way we craft ourself and ourselves–always in-the-world, of-the-world, with-the-world.

CITIZENSHIP

Citizenship is a social station; one who is addressed by the world can respond by engaging-the-world; citizen is one type of such engagement. Revolutionary, criminal, and politician are other stations for world-engagement and other forms of citizen. Young people in our studies rarely conceived of themselves as a citizen, even when explicit about wanting to "make the world better," i.e., help their neighborhood, families, and friends. Rarely did they talk about their work as political. Instead, they used the languages of helping and fixing as if what they were engaged in was a type of human service and/or God's work. Fixing was their metaphor for making it better. Even more rarely did young people explicitly use the language of prevention, although the idea was often present in their purpose, including control as a preventive strategy, for example, keep the situation from getting worse, get it under control, make it safe for kids. All are preventive levels, primary to tertiary.

In an evaluative perspective, the absence of explicit citizen language and the presence of the helping and fixing metaphors show that these young people either were not taught to name their work as civic engagement, public work, citizenship or citizen work and/or they simply did not speak this way to us. After four years and hundreds of interviews, we suspect the former: There was little systematic teaching or mastery of a civic paradigm of youth (and adult) activism.

Without such a theory, model, or language, the young people were left to the everyday languages of school, friends, family, religious group, community, and those of the larger public world. Here is the likely source of their conceptualization of their work and their ways of talking about it as forms of caring (Mayerhoff, 1971)–helping and fixing. In their usage, caring is good and it is what family and friends are about and, for some, it is a way to understand their God–as caring about them, their family, friends, and about the world: A benevolent, caring, attentive, and aware God.

God-talk (MacQuarrie, 1967) has a venerated place in the theology and practicalities of vocation for, in some conceptions, it is God who calls us to our earthly work and, through this, to our place-in-the-everyday and to our true, authentic, meaningful, and responsible self. In one tradition, this is reversed and it is Human Being who in work invites the presence of the Eternal Other: do good work and do it right, especially with others, and that constitutes the invitation for God to be present (Friedman, 1991). Naming one's work and one's self in theological, spiritual, or God-terms fits with a vocational understanding of self. And it can fit with an understanding of self as citizen. No young person named the work in this way in this study. We did hear this in another study of vocation with young people (Richter, Magnuson, & Baizerman, 1998). If God was spoken about, it was in the context of church and there was no connection stated joining church work to non-church citizen-work or to citizenship within one's congregation. To us, the latter is powerfully true, especially among young people active in their congregations. They were trained citizens in and of their religious and spiritual community. There they learned to do community work and many easily transferred this theory, language, skills, and citizen orientation to their PA efforts.

Those who did not think or talk in God-theological-religious language games spoke about caring, helping, and fixing in secular tones. They too usually had a larger conception, even philosophy, of their work not unlike their religious and church-attending peers. But theirs was most often a philosophy close to therapy: To care and to help is to make it better; this will make us feel better, be freer in how we do our lives (because the bad stuff is gone), and be and feel responsible because "we are doing our part to make things better."

Inside the base of both secular and religious conceptions, the young people hold typically implicit models of community, responsible self and a public, active self–*homo politicus*, *homo civicus*, citizen: citizen is their way of "making a difference" in their near world. This is their calling; the world in its pain, tumult, anger and unfairness addresses them. And through PA they learn to respond and practice their response. In this they are also practicing the living of a vocational identity–me as citizen.

PA in schools and community centers comes to be a world, a subculture of guided youth activism, a space for exploring and trying and reflecting on ways of being oneself, on how to be me. PA can become a life-style enclave, a space where citizen comes to be and to mean a certain kind of person who sees herself in certain typical ways and has a particular look with certain dress, music, chemical use, hairstyle and other beliefs and actions. PA had hoped to create in these settings a new culture of citizen and public worker, and indeed it had in several small Catholic schools in Minnesota and Missouri. There the PA subculture came to be a dominant school culture, at it did also in one Kansas City, Missouri, community center. In an evaluation perspective, PA failed in this transformative effort for, we believe, theoretical and practical reasons detailed in part in our evaluation reports (Hildreth, Baizerman, & VeLure Roholt, 2001; VeLure Roholt, Hildreth, & Baizerman, 2003). Yet this goal remains worthy, if likely unachievable, in large, complex urban middle and high schools, not because of the quality of the idea but precisely because of the nature of the setting as such–its structure and how it is run by school districts and building principals. In this failure to institutionalize and diffuse PA is its failure to achieve its laudable goals of changing civics education so as to better prepare young people for life-long active citizen work. PA remains a better and more effective way to show the citizen vocation to young people than any passive civics education curriculum. But to date it has failed to gain long-term, effective presence in all but a few school systems, here in the U.S. (Minnesota, Kansas, Missouri) or internationally (Northern Ireland, Palestine, Turkey). And this is too bad.

In contrast, there is a large, growing and effective social movement to make service learning required in American public and private schools, colleges, and universities. Service learning integrates service projects into formal classroom instruction, using the service experience as another tool for teaching required curriculum (Waterman, 1997). This strategy can also be read through the lens of vocation. In these initiatives, young people typically spend a few hours a week in doing tasks in a real world setting. This provides opportunity for youth to explore new places, activities, and people, making these and themselves available for guided reflection and other learning approaches. Here too young people are in spaces where they may be addressed by the world and hear a vocational call. Typically, service learning is not political, i.e., mostly about power, group interests, public policy, although it may be (Boyte, 1991). Rather, it has a more human service tone in practice, with politics placed within a frame of needed services. At most, it is reformist, as expected, given its auspice and location in schools. Many, many students hear a calling to "make a difference" and/or to "make things better" during or after their involvement in service-learning projects.

A vocation reading clarifies the most common answer young people (and adults) give as to why they participate in PA (and similar activities and in certain professions), and it contributes too to a grasp of the notion and social role citizen; It also adds value to understanding the social value of civic duty.

CIVIC DUTY

Civic duty means simply the individual's responsibility to her or his member communities–where one lives, works, goes for spiritual sustenance, plays, resides, and to the larger proximate and distal governmental and other political entities at all of these sites. It is one's responsibility to the communal. Civic duty broadly put is a social obligation in our society, one expected to be experienced and felt as a personal responsibility–to be informed about larger social and everyday public issues, to reflect and form opinions on these, to consider and to act on behalf of self and others. Civic duty is attached to the social role, the station in life, citizen. To be called to "make the world better," to "make a difference" in the public sphere is to be and to do citizen. A vocational reading makes clear the synaptic connections between and among civic duty, citizen, personal responsibility, and that praxis called citizenship: The individual is joined to God and to world in good work.

BECOMING INVOLVED; STAYING INVOLVED

Exploration of the discourses, "I want to make a difference" showed it to be a motive-term, purposive, and self-directional, specifically, about one's compelling commitment to "do something" for self and others both, something with meaning to self and others and to do this act or action in a socio-political realm. We looked briefly at this phrase through the lenses of accounts, reasons, explanations, and understanding of cause: How do we understand this young person in PA who decided/chose to take-on a public issue? Now we add to the taking-on of an issue, continuing to work on it: Why do young people stay in PA?

The simple, correct, and partially complete answer is that once taken on in school as school work, credit bearing or not, and once one's schedule includes this class (involvement, project, service-learning), it is difficult and disruptive to get out of it; in many schools and at both the middle and high school levels, opting-out is neither a simple nor supported act: Once in, one is typically in for the duration–a semester usually–rarely a year. Some students sign-up for PA term after term, sometimes over 2-3 years. In some schools in Missouri and Minnesota, especially small Catholic ones, all students must participate every term of their school career, even in one school, beginning in kindergarten. Leaving aside those who were required to participate every semester, why do students join and stay in PA? Does their answer, "I want to make a difference" convince us that it is true and sufficient to explain their decisions?

Students join because they have to (a school required course or experience) or choose voluntarily to belong. Why choose this? Because their friends are involved, siblings did it and liked it, the teacher is cool, the other classes are "boring," and/or this is "real life." "I can be in the same class/group as students from other grades." "I like this boy or girl who signed-up." "My mom says that I have to." "It is something that will look good on my application to (high school, college, a scholarship, etc.). "I want to make a difference in my school and/or community." We looked at this last phrase in the context of the front-end decision to become involved; here note that this is in contest with these many other reasons for deciding/choosing to get involved. We take a few more strands implicit in the youth claim of involvement and unwind and examine these.

Wanting to make a difference, seeing opportunity to do so, and acting on this are all implicit in the claim; so too is knowing what and how to do something positive. It cannot be assumed that middle and high school students in the United States know much about any of this; this is not typical of civic education curricula–theoretical or experiential. Some youth learn this through church involvement, others from parents involved in community action and/or professional work and, for a very few, by participating in school government or youth organizations. While there is much about this that is commonsense, in the sociocultural sense of folk wisdom and in common citizen knowledge, there is far more that is unique knowledge about and knowledge how to. These require mastery, education, training, coaching, and mentoring. Citizen work is craft work and in schools, neighborhoods, and groups, it is particularistic and contextualized ways of thinking and acting, alone and, more typically, in groups. Wanting to make a positive difference must become mastering the ways of thinking, doing, and being basic to socio-political activism in school, group, and community. It means that stopping violence or the abuse of children or neighborhood drug dealing must become *how* to do this–the options and possible actions, knowledge, skills and attitudes basic to democratic, non-violent, just, and equitable collective social change efforts. When civic training is done well, as it often is in PA, and the young people believe they are learning real and useful stuff, they are more likely to become really involved, thus concretizing their typically more vague interests and goals, resulting in deeper commitment to the issue and to being and doing citizen: "I really want to make a difference" and "I'm learning how to do this (in my school, neighborhood or city; on this and that issue)."

Staying involved, young people say, has to do with both a sense of personal efficacy and social effect. They begin the process of social change–the work–and working on "the work," which reinforces their commitment both to the issue and to the process. They may change issues but they hold steady on wanting to "do something positive." Action as such, more than incremental gains on their issue, seems to be the source of their continued involvement; involvement and participation become engaged-ment: they become hooked to the work and, with it, to hope and the possibility of truly "making a difference." Action begets continued involvement. Doing something works to keep them wanting to "do something to make a difference."

Young people stay involved because they are "doing something" and this contrasts directly and decisively with the rest of school where they "just sit, listen, tune-out, take notes," send text-messages or nap: action is real. From the cellular to the political levels, to do is to be, especially so in the United States. Through action they name themselves and are named by others, and both namings are outside the typical student culture's social worlds of skateboarder, hick, jock, stoner, geek, motorhead, preppy, and the like. Unlike those terms and those youth, they are now activists, typically a small and marginalized world in most United States public and private (and religious) schools. In this they have achieved uniqueness in a school world which both invites and denounces this; being different and fitting in are both especially strong values there, and these are often in conflict, more rarely mutually supportive in particular spaces and moments.

The activists call for appointments and often meet adults in their school building or at school headquarters and also in city government–politicians and functionaries. Young people may contact public media, from community newspapers to local television news, and business people, from the corner store to the local factory and the bank and insurance company: they are doing "real stuff" in the "real world."

Youth stay with this work because they are working–doing something–and that doing puts them in the adult world in new ways–as a player–on issues that matter to youth and often to adults. This is not, "What are you wearing to school?" or "Did you hear about Juanita?" but real stuff, i.e., adult stuff. This is a chance to be grown-up. This we and they take as the core source of their continuing involvement. This is heady stuff, where their response to the call or address of an issue brings young people into experiences of responsible action while acting like older youth, even adult-like, and feeling older and more mature than before and more grown-up than their friends and age-peers. Making a difference is being grown-up. The vocational call to citizen engagement is a way of being mature and doing good both and at the same time.

READING VOCATION THROUGH YOUTH CIVIC ENGAGEMENT

Up to now, we have read YCE through the lens of vocation. Here we read in the other direction to learn what YCE illuminates about vocation and the vocational. There is a useful distinction between the traditional understanding of vocation in theology and sociology and of vocational as understood in theology, sociology, and education: as presence in the lives of young people without necessarily carrying the notion of higher being. To watch young people doing civic work in their school and community and to listen to them talk about this in one-on-one and small group interviews is to take seriously their claim that the work and PA is to them real and meaningful and that they expect it to have consequence on the world–friends, family, neighborhood–and on themselves. To them the experience is authentic, responsible and transcendent, themes identified by Magnuson (1999) as basic to vocation; it appears this way to the three of us, in most cases. Accepting their claim as true that they find themselves in compelling commitment to "make a (positive) difference" in their worlds, they seem to be and they sound as if they are indeed individuals with a calling, living a calling, living in response to a world-address. Does this in any way make them different than if they were simply involved, participating, being political? What comes along with the vocational that makes them and their work in some way different, and what about this illuminates our interest in vocation and the vocational?

A young person who seems, sounds, and is living vocationally is relatively easy to discern and relatively hard to describe in the language-worlds of social and behavioral sciences but far easier to do so in poetic, spiritual, or philosophical languages. They seem integrated, holistic, and purposive, and they speak about their work as making them more fully a part of their world. While only a very few youth used the words calling or vocation(al) most who were offered definitions said that these terms caught what it was like to be them doing and being themselves in this work. At minimum, the notion and the meanings of vocation have resonance and utility for naming a particular kind of self, one engaged in something larger than personal interest, something public or civic. Moreover, these terms give a particular shape and form to this mode-of-being and doing self, one which attends to the personal and to the social simultaneously, if you will, one interpenetrating the other. In most Western and Northern conceptions of the self, the world is background, or partially incorporated in self or in the form self-in-the-world (of everyday life), co-present, that is, self is embedded in life always and always this embeddedness is in everyday life. In some individuals, the vocational, God, and world are co-present while, for others, world-address and self-in/through response are core: in both, the religious and the secular (or the differently religious) *require* the "and"–always both, always together. The self is less than the vocational self, and the vocational citizen self is a more complex character than either the social role citizen self or the just the citizen self. This complexity is presumed good because the vocational brings with it the possibility of a particular type of individual internal dialogue–between the secular and the sacred, between different configurations of the secular-sacred, and between the reflective self and the lived-being on topics such as "What do I believe? What do I stand for? What compels me to act publicly? Who am I? These are perennial self-interrogatives: What do I believe? What will I defend? How should I live my life? What should I do in this situation? This type of self reflection is said to have particular salience during adolescence but, obviously, these are pertinent and defining questions over the whole of the life-course. Moving from the scientific developmental to the sociopolitical, these interrogatories are far deeper, more penetrating and, arguably, at least as relevant as those about citizenship in the typical middle and high school civics curriculum. These can be used to get at the moral basis of democratic citizenship and citizen work as well as the moral basis of individual living and being in community. YCE brings vocational into these conversations.

YCE makes vocation a practical, everyday frame of analysis for citizenship, the life-station and, for citizen, the self.

REFERENCES

Bellah, R. (1986). Habits of the heart: Individualism and commitment in American life. Berkeley: University of California Press.

Boyte, H. (1991). Community service and civic education. *Phi Delta Kappan, 72*(10), 765-767.

Boyte, H., & Skelton, N. (1997). The legacy of public work: Education for citizenship. *Educational Leadership, 54*(5), 12-18.

Cresswell, T. (2004). Place: A short introduction. Malden, MA: Blackwell Publishing.

Farr, J., & Boyte, H. (1997). The work of citizenship and the problem of service-learning. In R. Battistoni & W. Hudson (Eds.). Experiencing citizenship: Concepts and models for service-learning in political science. Washington, DC: American Association for Higher Education.

Friedman, M. (1991). Encounter on a narrow ridge: A life of Martin Buber. New York: Paragon House.

Gerth, H. H., & Mills, C. W. (1958). From *Max Weber*: Essays in sociology. New York: Oxford University Press.

Hildreth, R., Baizerman, M., & VeLure Roholt, R. (2001). Major findings year 2 of public achievement evaluation. Retrieved April 27, 2007, from http://www.publicachievement.org/pdf/evaluations/report2000-1.pdf

Lyman, S., & Scott, M. (1970). Sociology of the absurd. New York: Appleton-Century-Crofts.

Macquarrie, J. (1967). God-talk: An examination of the language and logic of theology. London: S.C.M. Press.

Magnuson, D. (1999). Social interdependence: The goal structure of moral experience. Ph.D. Dissertation, University of Minnesota.

Mayeroff, M. (1971). On caring. New York: HarperCollins Publishers.

Mills, C. W. (1963). Power, politics, and people: The collected essays of C. Wright Mills. New York: Oxford University Press.

Richter, D., Magnuson, D., & Baizerman, M. (1998). Reconceiving youth ministry. *Religious Education, 93*(3), 340-357.

Spelman, E. (2002). Repair: The impulse to restore in a fragile world. Boston: Beacon Press.

Tilly, C. (2006). Why? What happens when people give reasons . . . and why. Princeton, NJ: Princeton University Press.

VeLure Roholt, R., Hildreth, R., & Baizerman, M. (2003). Year four evaluation of Public Achievement: Examining young people's experiences or Public Achievement. Retrieved April 27, 2007, from http://www.publicachievement.org/pdf/evaluations/report2002-03.pdf

Waterman, A. (Ed.). (1997). Service-learning: Applications from the research. Mahwah, NJ: Lawrence Erlbaum Associates, Publishers.

The "Youth" in Youth Civic Engagement

Youth civic engagement (YCE) is ostensibly about youth–adolescents, teenagers, young people, students–in some of the many scientific and everyday words used to name and categorize persons who are chronologically *about* 12-22 years old. Because youth civic engagement is about young people, at least in part, we explore here this obvious, taken-for-granted but, ultimately, complex notion. This is done by reading YCE through the lens of youth and reading youth through the lens of YCE. Throughout, we use data from our study of Public Achievement (PA) in the United States (Kansas, Missouri, Minnesota, and Wisconsin), in Northern Ireland and, in this chapter, from Palestine (Gaza and the West Bank), where it is called Popular Achievement.

READING YCE THROUGH THE LENS OF YOUTH

Is YCE really about youth and young people? It depends on who you ask. To its founder, Harry Boyte, and to many political activist and political theorists, PA in particular and YCE in general are about democracy, civic life, and citizenship in the future and (almost less so) in the present. It is about preparing young people to be reflective, nonviolent, just and active life-long citizens in their community and country. This is the classic notion of youth (youthhood) as a time of "preparation" for "real-life" and adulthood. Later we examine whether this so-called "psychosocial moratorium," which is presented as a "developmental" imperative or need, that is, genetically and biologically driven, is indeed this or whether instead this is a perspective or, better, an ideology that supports a particular conception of the life-course (not the life-cycle), as institutionalized in the United States and in much of the West and North.

This conception of adolescence and youthhood too easily misses the crucial developmental, sociopolitical and personal importance for young people of viable, authentic, meaningful and efficacious involvement now, during their youth, for both their current and future well-being and for the well-being of community and polity.

Notice that in the previous paragraph we added the present to the future and added the presumptive value of participation to the young person, not only to citizen politics, civic society and democracy. It is precisely this interest in youth as such which is not found in the work of most political activists and theoreticians (while it is seen at times political science research); there is some attention by writers in these traditions to youth activism and youth social movements, that is, group political action in the present, with youth *as* youth. To those interested in young people, there is a substantial literature on their activism and civic engagement, from both social change and educational perspectives. Much depends on the author's conception of youth.

WHAT IS "YOUTH"?

There are several everyday words for those aged 12-22 years: youth, adolescent, young person, teenager, student and employee, for example. Each is used in everyday talk and some are also in scientific discourse where they also have technical meanings. There are many language-games for the use of these terms–everyday and technical and the many different spheres of the everyday–family, friends, neighborhood, school, health, and the like, and to make this even more complex, there are also many different technical domains such as medicine, education, employment, and justice in which these words about young people take on specific meaning and their own rules for use.

Below these words and their everyday and technical uses are two basic, different, yet complementary sociocultural, political, economic, and scientific conceptions of this chronological age and of persons of age: One is biogenetic and the other is broadly social. In the United States, in general, and in the academy and the helping professions, the dominant paradigm is development and age (Baars, Hendricks, & Visser, 2007). The former is the overarching theory of human growth driven by human population and individual genetics (and thus biology, neurology, biochemistry, and the like) in social context and the latter is a unit of measure, typically in years; individuals live chronological age and are assessed to be a developmental age. This biogenetic model of human being over its life-span is biologically reductive, natural, that is, "the way things are" in nature, and our "best science." Typically, this scientific model names persons in the chronological age-range 12-19 as adolescents and frames them in bio-psycho-social terms as adolescents. Such individuals are understood as located in a life-cycle, itself divided into "stages," one of which is adolescence, which is subdivided into early, middle and late. The body, cognitive structure and function, personality and even social behavior are, broadly speaking, attributed to "development" and, in the hands of its best practitioners, to development-in-context of history, place, society, culture, family, neighborhood, friends, and other people, institutions and realities of the near to far environment.

The second broad perspective on this chronological age begins with this social and cultural context and seeks to understand how it works locally to globally to create and use age-groups and so-called traits or characteristics said to be typical of individuals whose bodies have been alive a certain length of time. Writing this last phrase as we did was intentional; to invite you to consider Hockey and James' (2003) anthropological insight that age is a way that society's mark the passage of time; that is, age is a social fact invented and used politically, culturally and socially as part of the way groups, communities and societies organize the socially constructed life-course (Gubrium, Holstein, & Buckholdt, 1994); that is, the biogenetically driven life-cycle of birth to death is given social form and social meaning: Infancy, childhood, (Jenks, 1996) and "old age" (Katz, 1996) are sociocultural, political, and economic categories used to make sense of natural biodevelopmental changes in individuals. Since time as such does not cause change (Lesko, 2001), the natural science model must explain these changes in other terms; this it does showing how chemical and other similar processes work. From this level, they move upwards to the cell and onwards to the individual and then to the age-group–youth. Biology is real; the developmental is a metaphoric organization of this. There is nothing "natural" about these categories, although it is interesting that such chronological age conceptions, while differing in specifics, seem to be quite consistent across history, place, and culture (Qvortrup, Bardy, Sgritta, & Wintersberger, 1994). There is less consistency about life-stages across history and society because of changes in economies, family-life, and the like.

In this second family of broad social conceptions of youth, primacy is given both to the local, i.e., around here or in that community (Cresswell, 2004), as well as to the societal. This is true for legal definitions, for example, the so-called "age of maturity" at 18 or 21 in general, with "legal age" depending on activity such as obtaining a driver's license, drinking alcohol in a pub, having the right to be married or the right to medical care without parental notification.

In its clearest forms, those who use these broadly sociopolitical and economic conceptions of the age category "youth" argue that while the biological is real, potent and consequential, it is in the social organization of these biological facts where youth is constructed as a meaningful social category and social reality, with real-world consequences for the society, this age-group as such, individuals of this age, and the relations between this age-group and other, e.g., adults (parents, teachers, police) and child (no longer a child; now a teenager). Let's now ground the philosophical and theoretical with an example from YCE.

The Developmental and Youth Civic Engagement

Using the bio-developmental model, YCE is about adolescents being taught in age-appropriate ways the knowledge, attitudes, and skills for life-long active citizenship, particularly about voting and keeping "informed" about civic issues. Given their stage of cognitive and related ethico-moral development, the most effective (i.e., proven) way to teach these is a, b and c. For example, given what is known about adolescence, it is likely to be more effective if the teaching is done in age-segregated peer groups, with adolescents chosen for groups based on their peer relationships within and outside the school. Learning should be organized in group settings, with intensity (time per week), duration (weeks in a year) taken into account (Eyler & Giles, 1999). What does the best developmental science say?

Scientific developmental reasons may be given as to why such an effort is important to the adolescent at this life-stage; social context may be added too, with a value statement on the importance of such preparation for the vitality of democracy. Note the obvious that the ideas of citizen and democracy, non-violence, and social justice and equity are social and personal values, and the applied development approach put its science in the service of these values and also in the service of a value-based conception of adolescent, indeed, of adolescent-in-the-context-of a democratic ideal.

Is there anything wrong with this, anything troubling about it? In one sense, not at all, because here is applied science being used in response to a meaningful social issue, and it is being used in ways in which the science serves the social value of citizen democracy. In another perspective, this approach is problematic in that its conceptions of adolescent need, competence, and healthy development are not value neutral, scientific terms. Rather they are value-laden and moral. If the applied development model of adolescent is itself a moral perspective as well as a scientific construct, then a model of YCE based in applied developmental science is another moral conception which must be read and taken as such and, as such, must compete on those terms with other such moral conceptions. That is, this is not about a scientifically proven and true model of adolescence and adolescent civic engagement versus a moral/value-based model, with the former taken as more potent because it is scientific. Rather it is about different moral conceptions, each seeking social, public and scholarly legitimacy by using different claims.

Another problem with the applied developmental approach is far less rational, indeed comes close to being heard as at least non-rational, if not irrational. We have trouble with the mechanical-like, the technological-like, aesthetic of this approach, its apparent orderliness and cleanliness with none of the subtlety, confusion, passion and variation that we find among persons, especially when they are seen as person-in-the-world-of-everyday life. In the tumult of the everyday, the science seems not only technological but also sterile, incomplete, simplistic, and, in effect but not in the intent of its practitioners, classist, racist, sexist, ahistorical, and simply naive. Indeed, if YCE is about broad conceptions of the civic, of politics, of citizen and of involvement, of participation and engagement, the applied perspective, model and technology is anything but when used in practice. It is adult truth in the service of adult goals, primarily. This is politics! It is about interests, power, and legitimacy.

All of this is in tension with the dream that science could be used effectively to "make society better" and individuals happier, less pained and more effective in their everyday lives. It is not the goal of science as such that we find troublesome but how it has too often been used as ideology and technology.

READING YCE THROUGH YOUTH

Applied development is grounded in a scientific conception of the young person as adolescent, and its approach to civic engagement is through this scientific construct. A contesting conception, youth, is broadly social, political, economic, and time/place-specific, focused on the now, the emergent and the future, adulthood and old age. In this frame, civic engagement has benefit now and later for both young person and community (civic life). Reading YCE through the lens of youth, it is clear at once that there are more flexible chronological age markers for this age-group in contrast to firmer and less flexible age-limits for the scientific adolescent. Second, scientific adolescence is a universal, while youth is time/place and population-bound: local, actual definition of youth counts most, and these are given by neighborhood, friend and group. To both conceptions, context matters, but differently. Youth is a context-based conception while adolescence is not. A third difference is that adolescence/adolescent are scientific terms and, as such, are presented as value-neutral, while youth is an explicitly social term and as such can not escape implicit and explicit valuational, moral, and socio-cultural meanings. Fourth, the applied scientific has an empirically proven technology for enhancing adolescent development in the social domain of civic life, while those working under the banner of "healthy youth development"–a moral frame with (applied) science overtones. Both use the same theory and research findings, with youth development practitioners adding in local flavor and realities. In contrast, those who are active in the civic and political realms see youth as workers (needing training and supervision) of a certain age, given in years: first worker, then age. Another typical reading of youth in that gaze is as member while others are activist, volunteer, and citizen. By referring to social role and not to birth age, these conceptions serve to highlight the place and contribution of the person over her body age. Of course, in the realities of a project and other life-contexts, age as such is usually embedded, e.g., student, young activist, student activist. In contrast to scientific developmental modes of reading and meaning where a particular age means a particular set of (likely) capacities, with youth in social roles, while the reality may be the same, it is perceived and spoken about programmatically as in having to train and supervise young workers in different ways than older workers. On the other side, these non-scientific perspectives emphasize "the positive" characteristic of "young people"–their inquisitiveness, energy, enthusiasm, commitment, passion, and perseverance, for example. Obviously, these too are age-graded and implicitly developmental but are treated as commonsense, as folk-knowledge, not as science, and thus these claim a different legitimacy.

YCE is about politics broadly put, and the knowledge, attitudes, and skills needed for effective social action for social change, on the scale local to international. Effective social activists of all ages learn and use these. Older activists have more opportunity to learn and use these. Those with more activist experience are likely better at this work than most beginners. Again, age and time show up as natural, real, and meaningful themes in YCE where these are treated as activities and tasks to be undertaken as in training and preparing workers. What most adult activists have more of than most youth activists is more experience (age/time) and more experiences of a certain type–activist experiences. The ideal adult activist has learned from involvements and is a more effective worker in, for example, running meetings, analyzing situations and problems, setting goals, imagining likely effective strategies, and the like. Most young people have fewer of these experiences, knowledge, and skills. Depending on the organization, initiative or project and its philosophy and practices, it may be decided that the more experienced must train, watch-over, and evaluate the beginners and the less able.

How to train youth to be civic activists, now and life-long? This is a pedagogical question that adolescent developmentalists work out using their science of learning. This is also basic in YCE. Indeed, in school-based initiatives such as PA in the US, in Northern Ireland and in some sites in Palestine, training-for and training-in civic engagement is the major effort. It is typically carried-out as experiential learning where the learning-about and the learning-how-to are joined to action on a group-decided project. Evaluation may also be an inextricable practice in this process, with the goal of improving practice to more likely and consistently meet project goals. In contrast, in adolescent development evaluation, focus is on change in the individual young person's developmental status, that is, cognition, moral reasoning, and also skill mastery. In youth civic engagement, the latter is also assessed. Under grantor pressure, distortion is very often brought to YCE in the requirement that evaluation include individual change read in developmental and school terms (e.g., grades, attendance) rather than in sociopolitical terms as effective worker. YCE has great interest also in changes in their participants, but their preferred focus is on their beliefs, understanding, and knowledge about democracy, citizenship, and citizen work. When this is assessed, as we and others have done (Hildreth, Baizerman, & VeLure Roholt, 2001; VeLure Roholt, Hildreth, & Baizerman, 2003), the results are clear: Most young people did not have a substantive grasp of these concepts and lived-realities before or after their involvement. We think this is because the projects did not focus on this and that the students were neither taught this material fully and systematically nor used it in their group or individual reflections. It is the very absence of this content, this rationale for the PA praxis, this democratic philosophy that opens the space for other overarching conceptions of the work and sources of legitimacy for it. One socially, culturally, and politically normative frame is "causing and helping" such as a human service language and way of making sense. Also available because it is part of school culture is the frame of "my friends"; "they're doing it and I want to be with them so I'll do it." A third school culture account is learning: "It seems interesting and I may learn from it, 'get something out of it.'" And, always, "I'll do it because it will look good on my college application." Just a reminder that these and other such accounts aside, participants may still come to understand, enjoy, even master citizen ways-of-being, continue their involvement on local public issues and, indeed, become life-long active citizens. This opens the evaluative question of whether young people who take on this mode of being called citizen but who do not have a civic account for their lived-actions are to be understood as showing a positive outcome of an YCE initiative. Is one a success only if she shows both action and (the correct) account?

From a different angle, reading YCE through the lens of youth and young people suggests that their most valid account may be the one that belongs to their world of meanings, whether or not it is what the project teaches and wants to hear back from them. It may be the most important insight of reading YCE through youth, youthhood, young people and YCE setting (e.g., school, youth club, community center) is that young people's frames and ways of making sense of their involvement may be in a different realm and in a different language than those who conceive, design, implement, manage, and evaluate actual YCE projects: they do it on adult terms and make sense of it on their terms. This is about "youth culture" and, more important, about site-specific youth subculture and life-style enclaves, and schools are a primary site of such youth worlds. Those closest to the participants typically know something, if not a lot, about these worlds and groups and their interpretative paradigms–how meaning is constructed, diffused, sustained and changed. They have much to tell about how YCE works in that space, as do the youth who are involved. They must be asked to make sense of YCE on their terms, as well as using those required by the sponsor, the site or the evaluators:

A duck by any other name. . . .

If it walks like a duck, quacks like a duck and eats like a duck. . . .

READING YOUTH THROUGH YCE

If reading YCE through a youth lens reminds us to pay attention to the young people and their ways of making and sustaining meaning and meaningfulness, reviewing this and reading youth through a YCE lens opens up the conceptions of youth, young person, youthhood, adolescent, student and worker. The two readings disclose related insights.

The ideal young person in YCE initiatives may be the adolescent, the scientific young person, who thinks and acts and lives as an adolescent, in ways laid-out in the scientific model of adolescence and found in empirical research on persons at this life-stage and with a certain chronological age: "She is like this and given what we want to accomplish with her, she is more likely to do it if we carry it out this way." This is an example of applied adolescent development. Such an approach would take into account, for example, the setting to be worked in, the adults employed there, and her peers.

Actual young people are not scientific adolescents; instead they are in and of everyday worlds, albeit embodied in ways made partially clear by developmental and related science, with brains that work in ways made partially clear. A recent court case legitimizes scientific findings about the adolescent brain (Boyd, 2006), challenging socio-moral notions of responsibility (Ortiz, 2004). In the end, however, it is in the particularities that YCE (and life) go on: these particular young people in this particular group in this particular school at this historical moment. To understand YCE in general is to first understand it in its particulars; to understand youth and young person, student and citizen, it is first to understand these social roles as a way for understanding individual persons.

In other words, adolescent is a scientific construct, an abstraction, a generalization applied to a particular class of persons or to an individual. Youth is a *social role*, the incumbent of which is an individual, actual young person. YCE is about both of these. The first insight from reading youth through YCE is to realize that there are three readings necessary:

- What does YCE disclose about youth, the social role and symbol, metaphor, representation?
- What does YCE disclose about being and doing oneself as a youth?
- What does YCE disclose about those individuals who see themselves and call themselves youth, young person, teen, student, and the rest?

Social Role

There are macro and micro levels here. On the macro level, youth as social role refers to ways of doing and being certain ages, typically 12-22 years. Youth is the carrying out and age-graded social expectations about thinking, feelings, talking, acting, dressing, playing and the rest. Social roles are space/time specific, so what a youth is and how "youth" is to be done must be grounded to place and history–here/ now: Baker High School, 2004; the Crow Nation, Montana, 1986, for example.

In this view, citizen is a social role subject to the same rules of specificity. So too student and worker, teacher and leader. YCE says that what it means to be a youth participant depends–on local specifications. There is no single, universal way to do youth or citizen or participant or youth leader. For example:

- Being in a PA group and meeting with the school principal about safety in the building
- Volunteering in a nursing home
- Being an Eagle Scout
- Taking your nephews fishing
- Voting in school elections

One YCE project in the U.S. was run out of a community center by someone active in a particular religious-political philosophy and church. Those who were youth and citizens in his initiative did this in ways far different than anywhere else we evaluated. Their conception of youth was one who will be taught, their conception of student was unquestioning learner, and their conception of citizen was doing what you were told to do. This is the easy to grasp insight, one almost commonsensical now. Less so is the next insight.

Being and Doing Oneself as Youth

If youth as such is a social category, individuals perform, carry-out, and take on these social expectations; they become the role in the theatrical, performative sense. What is the experience and meaning to self and others of being and doing oneself as youth? (as student, a teenager, etc.). When I do youth. When I (do) (am) citizen. This perspective attends to the person *doing* the social role and, related, being the social role and, more radically, being who one is–herself. This is not just we are our roles but is, since we may be our many roles (some more than others), there is not a single me, but instead I am many.

How I do/am youth in one time/place setting may seem to fit or not with how I am/do youth in another. So too with citizen. And I may seem different being/doing student than being/doing citizen, worker, and youth. This is the self in post-modernity (Schrag, 1997). And this is a conception of person/self/being that is radically discontinuous with the older views of the self–the single unitary self. In earlier times, there was said to be a tighter, even better, fit between and among the social roles one took and one's self. The self then was seen as unitary then, now to the postmodernist, it is multiple (Schrag, 1997).

In practical terms, "bad kids" can take on and do great citizen work for their neighborhood; students with poor grades who have trouble with class readings may read civic engagement materials with less difficultly: Same kid, same brain, different world–different kid, as it were–to some extent. We interviewed many young people who found little value in school, goofed-off and screwed around and were taken and treated as problems, yet who flourished in an YCE initiative. This is an old story but one worth remembering as experiential learning programs become less available, more restrictive in admission and for the academic and behavioral elite, while the others work on basics. Not to be lost is whether and how YCE can be differently meaningful and powerful for many young persons as a way to do and be a youth. YCE is a good opportunity to explore worlds and, in so doing, explore how to name and then live-out one's self and also to integrate these selves into a dominant identity and personality. YCE can be such a field of exploration and play in the crafting of self (Melucci, 1996).

Youth and Others

To call oneself a youth, to experience one's body, time/space and others in this way is to be and to do youth. In the social world of others, they have to accept these performances if they are to see, react, and relate to that person as a young person, as a youth. What they think and what and how they act on that basis matters to that person, to them in their mutual worlds, and to the larger social order. This general point becomes particularly important in the context of school and in other social environments where age expectations are clear, patrolled and, if violated, challenged: *Act your age!* is not only the title of a very good book (Lesko, 2001), it is also a raw and tough sociomoral reminder to stay in one's appropriate age-role. Another common phase and book title is *How Old are You?* (Chudacoff, 1989), the two phrases (and books) show how chronological age is part of many social roles.

The insight is seen best in the case of citizen, the social role. In the sociolegal realm, citizen is specified by age as in the case of voting and criminal (juvenile) law; there is a minimum for the former and both minimum and maximum ages for the latter. Beyond that, little about citizen is age-specific. Could it be that it is this very absence of age referents contributes to adults not inviting young people into the citizen role, with some small exceptions, in schools, religious congregations, and neighborhood groups and clubs? Leadership in these is typically age-segregated, with youth excluded. No wonder youth is thought to need preparation; they are kept from the everyday and specialized learning that would come from their everyday involvement. A remedy? Train them. Another remedy? Involve them in authentic, meaningful and viable ways in the full spectrum of the community's everyday sociopolitical life. Why does this seem an odd idea to adults? In part because a younger chronological age means less experience, means less wisdom, means not yet ready. Inextricably part of all of this is youth as image–the teenager, the adolescent, not yet with capacity to take on such serious work, the work of communal living, public work–citizen. This thinking about youth is often not self-aware, because youth–the symbol, image, representation, metaphor–is so deeply in sociocultural, political and economic language and imagery that it is taken-for-granted and treated as natural (Baizerman, 1998; Lesko, 2001).

Making the exclusion of young people an even more powerful argument is recent biophysiological research and court rulings citing it on the adolescent brain and its capacities and limitations, such as high level reasoning and decision-making (Boyd, 2006).

Another View

YCE offers a direct and potent challenge to this perspective on and line of reasoning about youth. Our evaluations show unequivocally that most young people, when invited to take on the substantive, meaningful, viable and real social role of citizen, do so with competence and integrity by being invited, supported, and supervised. We have found that young people in school can cross age-graded, sex-specific role expectations and carry out the citizen role, not only in age-appropriate ways but, more importantly, in role-appropriate ways. They do citizen as a citizen would, not as a youth would! The exclusion of young people from citizen roles is not natural, nor is it based on a natural or a biochemical or neurological fact: exclusion is a sociopolitical decision and act, which at times use the natural, the biophysiological, the developmental as a moral account for this exclusion.

The history of the idea of youth (Mitterauer, 1986) and of young people (Levi & Schmitt, 1997) is the documentation of their increasing marginalization from their community's everyday life to a age-population segregated into age-specific ghettos such as schools, sport and recreation clubs, youth programs and the like. The misuse of folk wisdom and developmental science provide the account: involvement must be age appropriate and meet the test of readiness. Activities are age-segregated, with a resulting age-homogeneity in most social institutions so that young people of the same age are found together. Then it is said that simply by looking, it is easy to see how alike they are. This is because they are at the same developmental stage, it is said. Could it be that people who are segregated together for very long periods come to look like and be like each other?

Youth and Others

YCE discloses limitations and distortions in the developmental science conception of adolescent (Morss, 1996) by showing that properly pre-pared and supervised young people can take on and perform the citizen role in ways thought not possible simply because of their age. Some examples:

- Young people at a private, urban school worked for three years to design and build a new school playground. This required them learning planning code and arguing their case with the mayor and city council. In the end, the research and data they presented could not be contested.
- Kindergarten students at a public urban school worked together to get more equipment for their playground and their elementary gym.
- Older young people at an urban public school used local media to get the city to clean-up a vacant lot in their neighborhood and then developed the lot into a park.

Not too long ago, it was generally believed than African-Americans did not have the capacity to do the same work as Asians or Caucasians; women could not do men's work. These and so many more examples of sociopolitical, economic, legal and everyday classism, racism, sexism and the rest show social exclusion. Is youth our new excluded population?

Many political regimes fear their young people and work at co-opting them in governmental youth movements (Heer, 1974), lest the youth get organized and become a political force in society and politics. In other societies, these sociopolitical processes of marginalization, segregation, and cooptation result in the fact that young people spend lots of time together, thus creating a market and a youth culture (Mallan & Pearce, 2003). Both work to support keeping young people out of the worker economy and in the consumer economy, resulting in freeing jobs for older workers (Mizen, 2004). Consumer economy works to create and sustain worlds in which young people look, act, and are youth. Once so perceived by adults, they are taken as too young and not yet ready for adult roles such as citizen. Around and around this goes, the evidence from YCE projects unknown, marginal, little used, essentially irrelevant to the larger issues about the state of youth, the condition of youth, the youth questions (Cohen, 1997).

CONCLUSION

Youth as idea, image, metaphor, symbol, and representation as well as population-group and individual is a complex term used and reduced in everyday life to a few simple meanings. The technical, the subtle, the different angels of understanding and the poetry of intentional, thoughtful and crafted use cannot be heard over the loudspeakers used by merchants and politicians, by experts in adolescence and adolescents, and their normal development and typical problems. Youth as a word may be little used among persons that age in self-referral or in referring to these age-groups or their generation. Youth in the end may be an adult term used by them to refer to them. But youthhood is a fact of social life, and developmental changes in body and brain are facts of biological life. More complicated is how these two perspectives work in tandem and in opposition. Current efforts at genetic level explanation, seen by some as biologically reductive, are gaining scientific support and are being used politically to categorize, marginalize, segregate and demonize adolescents, youth and young persons. This use is demagogic, although most of its practitioners are seemingly well-meaning, seeking to better the condition of youth, to support their "full flourishing" and to prepare them for full, vital and viable roles as adults and citizens.

YCE as a praxis challenges dogmatic assertions based in science, philosophy, politics or folk wisdom that young people do not have the capacity or are unable or are unwilling to take on substantive social roles while they are and are seen as youth–as persons 12-22 years old and as young people. They indeed have the capacity, ability and willingness to be citizens now and into their adulthood and old age. YCE discloses these facts and supports them with anecdote and other narrative evidence.

Who wants to listen?

REFERENCES

Baars, J., Hendricks, J., & Visser, H. (Eds.) (2007). *Aging and time: Multidisciplinary perspectives.* Amityville, NY: Baywood Publishing Company.

Baizerman, M. (1998). It's only "human nature": Revisiting the denaturalization ofadolescence. *Child & Youth Care Forum, 28*(6), 437-444.

Boyd, R. (2006, December 19). Teenage trouble? Blame it on their brains. *Star Tribune.* Retrieved December 19, 2006, from http://www.startribune.com.

Chudacoff, H. (1989). *How old are you? Age consciousness in American culture.* Princeton, NJ: Princeton University Press.

Cohen, P. (1997). *Rethinking the youth question: Education, labour and cultural studies.* London: MacMillan Press, LTD.

Cresswell, T. (2004). *Place: A short introduction.* Malden, MA: Blackwell Publishing.

Eyler, J., & D. Giles. (1999). *Where's the learning in service-learning?* San Francisco: Jossey-Bass.

Gubrium, J., Holstein, J., & Buckholdt, D. (1994). *Constructing the life course.* Dix Hills, NY: General Hall, Inc.

Heer, F. (1974). *Challenge of youth.* Tuscaloosa,University, AL: The University of Alabama Press.

Hildreth, R., Baizerman, M., & VeLure Roholt, R. (2001). *Major findings year 2 of public achievement evaluation.* Retrieved April 27, 2007, from http://www. publicachievement.org/pdf/evaluations/report2000-1.pdf

Hockey, J., & James, A. (2003). *Social identities across the life course.* New York: Palgrave MacMillan.

Jenks, C. (1996). *Childhood.* London: Routledge.

Katz, S. (1996). *Disciplining old age: The formation of gerontological knowledge.* Charlottesville, VA: University Press of Virginia.

Lesko, N. (2001). *Act your age! A cultural construction of adolescence.* New York: Routledge Falmer.

Levi, G., & Schmitt, J. (1997). *A history of young people (Vol. 1 & 2).* Cambridge, MA: The Belknap Press of Harvard University Press.

Mallan, K., & Pearce, S. (2003). *Youth cultures: Texts, images, and identities.* Westport, CT: Praeger.

Melucci, A. (1996). *The playing self: Person and meaning in the planetary society.* Cambridge, UK: Cambridge University Press.

Mitterauer, M. (1986). *A history of youth.* Oxford, UK: Blackwell Publishers.

Mizen, P. (2004). *The changing state of youth.* New York: Palgrave MacMillan.

Morss, J. (1996). *Growing critical: Alternatives to developmental psychology.* New York: Routledge.

Qvortrup, J., Bardy, M., Sgritta, G., & Wintersberger, H. (Eds.) (1994). *Childhood matters: Social theory, practice and politics.* Aldershot, UK: Avebury, Ashgate Publishing Limited.

Ricoeur, P. (1991). *From text to action: Essays in hermeneutics, II.* Evanston, IL: Northwestern University Press.

Schrag, C. (1997). *The self after postmodernity.* New Haven, CT: Yale University Press.

Velure Roholt, R. (2006). *Democratic civic practice: Building democratic communities together. A training curriculum.* Belfast, Northern Ireland: Public Achievement Northern Ireland.

VeLure Roholt, R., Hildreth, R., & Baizerman, M. (2003). *Year four evaluation of Public Achievement: Examining young people's experiences or Public Achievement.* Retrieved April 27, 2007, from http://www.publicachievement.org/pdf/evaluations/report2002-03.pdf

Civic Youth Work

In the past few sections of this volume, we have four readings of Public Achievement (PA), Youth in Government (YIG), and the Youth Science Center (YSC). Each reading comes from the perspective of a particular theoretical frame–education, political theory, vocation, and youth. These four readings are designed both to illuminate and interrogate the programs in particular and youth civic engagement (YCE) in general. In the broadest sense, each program looks different when viewed from a different frame. But theoretical frames are more than simply shifts in perspective. Theories represent ways of organizing categories, scientific findings, and moral values. They help determine what counts as real and what does not. These frames matter because they are implicit in funding processes and expected educational outcomes such as, in the U.S., No Child Left Behind. We certainly believe in having clear expectations but want youth workers to be aware that behind these outcomes are theoretical frames that have real world consequences for practice. For instance, scientific discourses on adolescence determine, in part, what a teacher, social worker, or police officer may think is possible for a 12-year-old girl to think, feel, and do. In these initiatives we have seen how youth often defy these age-grade expectations, tackling complex issues that supposedly require a higher levels of moral, emotional and cognitive development.

The first part of this chapter summarizes each theoretical frame and distill three key ideas from our theoretical readings, and we distill three key ideas from our theoretical readings that we think are innovative. Then we translate theory into a new orientation to practice–*civic youth work*.

REVIEW OF FOUR THEORETICAL FRAMES

In chapter 7 we interpreted the three initiatives through the frame of education. Here, we contrast civic education with civic engagement. Civic education relies on standard definitions of citizenship and therefore focuses on learning content (knowledge *about* political institutions, principles, and processes of governance), mastering specific democratic skills (e.g., public speaking, critical thinking, etc.), and the attaining of particular dispositions (e.g., social responsibility, tolerance, compassion, etc.) (Butts, 1980; Patrick, 1996). Youth civic engagement challenges these conceptions of civic education. Rather than learning and knowing-about in order be better informed, it emphasizes learning through doing. There is a key shift from the future orientation of civic education–learning about in order to–to the present orientation of civic engagement–learning through.

This conception of YCE clearly resonates with and is situated in the larger literature on experiential education. Experiential education is more, however, than simply learning through doing. Even though we are learning (and not learning) all the time in the course of our everyday lives, experiential education represents the reconstruction of experience in ways that promote learning and growth. In academic terms, this expands learning through doing to *reflexive doing*–that is, the intentional and reflective practice. From our conversations with young people, we identified presenting an invitation, supporting democratic ways of working together, doing *real world* public work, and reflection as critical components to powerful civic learning experiences. In this sense, these three initiatives were philosophically and pedagogically experiential education (Dewey, 1938; Joplin, 1995; Kolb, 1984). They do not offer an alternative conception of experiential education but, rather, refine key principles towards civic engagement.

Chapter 8 was written from the frame of political theory. Here, we contrasted standard accounts of citizenship with our expanded alternative understanding of *lived citizen*. Standard accounts of citizenship focus on what citizens are (legal status), what they should *do* (desirable activity), and *how* they identify as citizens (collective identity). Translated into civic practice, this frame directs practitioners and researchers to the development of civic and political knowledge, attitudes, skills, and dispositions. Indicators of "positive" civic engagement include voting, volunteering, contacting public officials, following politics in the news, engaging in boycotts and the like. While each of these indicators are important parts of citizenship, this frame may not *count* many of the students in PA and YSC as civically engaged. Standard measures do not map onto programs in which young people have the freedom to co-create the activities, projects, processes and outcomes.

From our reading of the lived experiences of young people in these three initiatives, we came to see that these standard accounts miss something very important–they miss the embedded, embodied, and dialectical relationship between *doing, being* and *becoming* citizen in specific contexts. Drawing from Hannah Arendt, we emphasize that politics should not be understood as limited to pre-defined activities or places but that politics take place wherever people act in concert for public purposes. In addition to curricular and co-curricular programs, Arendt helps us see how museums, youth clubs, churches, and even families are possible places for engagement! Because these spaces for engagement do not arise spontaneously, we argue that an important part of YCE is to offer an invitation to engagement. We then turn to John Dewey to emphasize the interactive nature of YCE. Dewey directs our attention to lived experience, how each moment is pregnant with possibilities for learning and democratic citizenship. Our conversations with young people revealed that something as mundane as making a phone call can be an important source of learning and even transformation for an individual. Our alternative understanding of citizenship represents a broadening and opening to current discourses of citizenship. It hopes to knit together a more grounded, embodied, and fluid understanding of the relationship between *doing* citizen activities (PA, YIG, and YSC), *becoming* citizen (learning through interaction), and *being* citizen. Taken together, we advance *lived citizen* as the embodiment and integration of doing, becoming and being citizen.

In Chapter 9 we read YCE through the lens of vocation. Vocation may seem like a strange turn given its association with religion (hearing the call of God) and technical training (vocational education). However, we draw from the deeper and venerable tradition of vocation, in its religious and secular senses, to emphasize the idea of address and response. In our everyday lives, we find ourselves addressed or confronted by certain persons, issues, situations, conditions and ideas that are compelling; they require us to answer, to respond. How we hear this address and respond is who we are. We define ourselves; we craft ourselves in our lived-response. In this sense, we author ourselves in action, one form of which is citizen: lived-self as lived-citizen.

We examine this idea by unpacking and interpreting the statement we heard again and again in our conversations with young people–"I want to make a difference in my community." This statement can be read in terms of motive (the reason why I do this) or as a ritualized trope (a bullshit answer that young people think adults want to hear, like "don't take drugs"). We believe this statement becomes richer and clearer when read in terms of vocation. "I want to make a difference" represents a moral sense of commitment of the whole person. The vocational represents a an internal dialogue between the secular and the sacred, between such important issues as what I believe, what I stand for, and what compels me to act publicly and, ultimately, who I am.

In Chapter 10 we examined YCE through the lens of youth. Here we contrast the applied developmental model of adolescence with our alternative of youth as a social idea. The developmental model advances adolescence as a scientific fact, defined by chronological age in terms of cognitive, emotional, and physiological development. Simply stated, this model holds that an individual is defined by chronological age, say a 12-year-old girl, and this age defines certain traits, that is, age-appropriate ways of thinking, feeling, and acting. Even if we are not familiar with the social and biological scientific literature on adolescence, this developmental model is present in schools and other social environments where age expectations are clear, patrolled and, if violated, challenged. We are familiar, perhaps all too familiar, with statements such as "Act your age!" or "How old are you?"

As an alternative, youth as a social idea represents the social, political, and moral organization of these biological facts. Here we emphasize that youth is context-based; what we expect from youth is different in different contexts. In one sense, youth take on different social roles. We expect different things of a teenager who is a *worker* at a fast food restaurant than a *student* in an Advanced Placement class. Like student and worker, citizen is also a social role. This role is often age-graded–youth are subject to a different set of laws, are not allowed to vote, and in general are seen to need training in order to take on the moral responsibilities of citizenship. But more than simply playing a different role (as citizen), YCE represents a shift and rupture of age and role-based expectations youth. Instead of seeing youth as *not yet ready* and therefore *in need of training*, YCE challenges assertions based in science, philosophy, politics or folk wisdom that young people do not have the capacity or are unable or unwilling to take on substantive social roles while they are and are seen as youth, as persons 12-22 years old, and as young people. The young people in these initiatives have proven that they have the capacity, ability, and willingness to be citizens now!

THREE INNOVATIVE IDEAS

Throughout this book we have referred to the idea of *lived citizen*. It represents an attempt to get at citizenship from the inside, that is, from the lived experiences of civic engagement. In an important sense lived-citizen integrates the political, educational, and vocational frames we have just reviewed. It also ruptures expectations of young people in terms of age-grade expectations. Here, we distill three ideas from our theoretical readings of YCE that we think are innovative and serve as the foundation for our discussion of civic youth work in the concluding chapter.

Open and Expansive Understandings of Citizenship and Politics

We described how standard definitions of citizenship and civic engagement defines in advance the behaviors, attitudes, activities, and outcomes that "count" as civic or political. Drawing on Arendt and Dewey, we call for expanding the definition of "the political" to include any situation where people work in concert for public ends. This pushes us away from seeing citizenship as an individual attribute and towards seeing it as a collective enterprise. It also pushes us away from seeing politics as only happening in governmental institutions. Citizenship can be conceived of as an interactive process between individuals and their environments. Any situation, say, meeting a school principal, is pregnant with civic and political potential. This does not mean that any gathering or any meeting with a principal is civic or political. Following theories of experiential education, we believe that there must be an invitation, support, and reflection to bring about powerful civic learning and engagement.

Hence, the idea of *lived citizen* approaches politics from the inside out. It starts with young peoples' everyday lived experiences and then they develop an understanding of "the political" through the process of reflective engagement. This idea radically opens up the domain of politics. However, does it strip "the political" of substantive content? Can we, in this frame, call anything we want political? Is not a street gang defending its "turf" an example of collective action for the public end of protecting its neighborhood? Rather than focusing on one correct definition, we suggest establishing procedural criteria to define the political. Following Boyte and Farr (1997), we suggest that a robust understanding of "the public" or publics offers guidance. It is a procedural in the sense that "the public" should not be defined in advance but through inquiry and in the context of youth's lives. There are relatively simple criteria to help youth think through the public dimensions of their work. Framed as questions, they include: Who does this problem affect? How does it affect them? Are there differing views about the nature of the problem? What are the negative consequences of this problem for the community? Who are the stakeholders (who has power in relation to this problem)? What kinds of projects or solutions will make the best impact? Who will they affect? Will they be lasting, public, and meaningful?

We believe that public criteria may actually require more of youth workers. Instead of implementing curriculum or organizing prescribed activities, youth workers need to be open to young people's worlds and be willing to work co-creatively.

Youth as Citizens Now

Building on this expansive sense of citizenship, our reading of YCE through the lens of youth as an idea calls for reconceptualizing youth as citizens now. When implicated in developmental conceptions of adolescence, YCE is often seen as preparation for future citizenship. Instead, we argue that citizen engagement represents an opportunity to disrupt or overcome age-grade and social role expectations for youth. Instead of envisioning youth as apathetic, youth as a problem, or youth as the future, we call for seeing youth as youth: as promise and possibility.

What does it mean to see youth as promise and possibility? On a simple level it means not pre-judging young people based on what they look like, how old they are, how they talk, how they carry themselves, what friends they have. On a deeper level it means embodying an invitation for co-creation with young people. In everyday terms, this means starting where they are and taking their ideas seriously. But it is more than a way of doing things with young people, it is a way of being (oneself) together with young people. This mode of being co-present with young people has the potential to invite, foster and witness young people's becoming (citizen).

Lived-Citizen as Vocation

Many discussions of citizenship and civic engagement focus on the role of citizen, that is, citizenship is one role among many–student, worker, sibling, friend and the like. We believe that vocation represents a more powerful way to articulate citizenship as a mode of being in the world. This is a more integrated, wholistic, and purposive understanding of citizenship–it is a relationship and dialogue between an individual and the world she lives in. When we are "living citizens" we hear the address of the world in public and political ways and we are compelled to respond. "I want to make a difference in my community" is transformed into "I cannot be myself if I don't make a difference when I see _____." This sense of self-as-citizen, citizen-as-self, is the ultimate goal of YCE. Rather than just focusing on what young people learn through a particular program, we believe we should also pay attention to what happens after the program is over. Vocation is one way to understand the ways in which young people become and be citizens beyond civic programming.

BEING AND DOING CIVIC YOUTH WORK

Young people are exhorted to become involved in civic issues while at the same time they are actively marginalized by adults–and peer pressure–from structures of participation in school, community, faith-worlds, sports, and family. And they are poorly, if at all, prepared for civic engagement and rarely supported in long-term involvement. Basic to this invitation, exclusion, and irrelevance is the assumption that they are neither interested in nor ready for responsible participation on important issues.

In contrast, our stance is in other places, a geography of rights and the spaces of democracy. In these, youth civic engagement is given in virtue of an individual's birth, not in virtue of his/her chronological or developmental readiness. This follows Jeffs (2001) and others in democratic theory (Boyte & Skelton, 1997). In this view, positive developmental outcomes, however defined and in whatever value frame, can be valuable concomitant results of active, viable, authentic, and meaningful youth engagement, but they are neither its purposes nor its goal. The right to participate as a birthright is what is in play and is what must be protected to preserve democracy, and this right is not age-graded, except for the very young, those with severe and persistent mental incapacities and the senile.

In many societies, young people come to engage in issues important to them by being recruited into existing political or social action youth-only or age-mixed groups, being pressed into joining such groups by other young people or adults, or by creating their own issue-specific groups, among other possibilities. Adults who recruit or pressure youth to be involved may be employed by a political party, an issue-group, a school or youth program. Typically, these adults have little training in how to work in democratic ways with youth in groups, while they may have training and experience in work with young people as recreation leaders, high school teachers, church leaders, and volunteers in youth organizations. Typically, youth who do this leadership work with other youth also have little training. One reason for the absence of this training is that there is no institutionalized worker role in most places oriented to democratic civic practice (VeLure Roholt, 2006). It is this we would like to propose.

Civic youth work is an embodied invitation to young people to become and to stay involved in civic issues important to them. Its craft orientation is to address young people–individually and in small and large groups–by being present, co-creating, and finding opportunities for viable, authentic, and meaningful engagement. Civic youth work can be practiced anywhere in the life-worlds of young people on the level of their everyday, ordinary existence in school, community, places of worship and recreation, and even at home.

Civic youth workers go about being this invitation and address by their presence in spaces available to young people and by their presence as invitation (Friedman, 1974; Friedman, 1983). There is here a geography of democratic opportunity that joins invitation to opportunity and availability: they are there where democratic work can be done together. Civic youth workers orient to young people as co-creators of ongoing democratic spaces wherein both act their right to be there together and to work together on common interests, privileging those of the young people.

The frame of the civic youth worker is existential, with an orientation in the moment, in emergence, and co-creation. In this way the civic youth worker co-creates democratic space and time and in so doing embodies democratic practice, discloses democracy, and teaches democratic practices and skills. Such work is an infinite game (Carse, 1986), ongoing, emergent, with a few rules but no conclusion, no winner or loser: ongoing, as is democracy.

This ongoing work is a process of connected instances, moments brought into existence by the workers intention and act-of-invitation, over and over again, never ending. This is a worker mode-of-being, not reducible only to knowledge, attitudes, and skills–the classical trilogy of professional practice–but to praxis which becomes integrated in being en-act-ed. The worker literally invites the young person to make real a possibility within which they then work together. This calls for the worker to imagine the possibilities of space potential in every moment and to imagine living in every space–to imagine that the worker's act right now, here, will invite opening which worker and youth can occupy and use. What is, is actually made into a future. After that moment the same is done again, ad infinitum. In this way, the worker is *doing democracy* with another.

An observer of this might see worker and young people "working together" or simply being together. Without the knowledge necessary to discern, to know how to tell what it is and tell if it is real and true, the outsider may not be able to know and to say that what is seen is democracy and citizen. The outsider has to be a connoisseur. She or he can tell what is seen and the experience of it, one's feelings and thoughts. Those participating can describe what it is like to do and be self while doing this with a youth worker and, likewise, tell their feelings and thoughts and the meanings of doing and being in this way. In this we are given access to living-citizen, to the existential reality of citizen.

Basic to the interior and exterior description of the work is language and the issue for us is, "What are the languages of lived-citizen and lived-democratic practice?" At minimum, in the democratic ethos, one language must be everyday talk, folk-talk, as it were. Then there is the talk of the issue and the talk of the self-at-work and in other modes of being. Sometimes there is a reading of this living-text (Ricoeur, 1991) in the languages of politics, political philosophy, and political theory. Each language is a frame that, when used to read and speak, changes the reality of what is seen and said. For example:

Every day talk: "Well, having kids trying to make a difference . . . cause there are probably tons of adults trying to make a difference in something, and like they don't think kids can do it, so then they're giving kids a chance to try and make a difference in our community."

Talk of the issue: "We first started out in budget cut issues. Our first issue was the library and why the library was closed from schools and why we couldn't check out books. So we wanted to get some money for that. But in the end it got so complicated, so then we went to textbooks. And we got a lot of info like everybody was suing [county] because they was getting more money for schools than [other suburban schools]. So we got some help. We knew if we did try to take it to the Supreme Court we would have had some back up."

Talk-of-the-self-at-work: "The whole entire group was sitting around and he was drawing on the board. We were talking about regular polygons. And we worked our way up, we were like, 'What's the word for a hundred-sided polygon?' And then we said, 'What's the name for an infinite-sided polygon?' and it was a circle. And I was just trying to think of what can you take and make it into a triangle and would transform into a circle. And I came back the next day and I said, 'What if we used a laser inside of a circular mirror and just bounce it around in there?'"

All of this matters if one goal of these youth civic engagement efforts is civic education: One may not know this is what is going on unless one know that this is what is going on: to name is to see, feel, make sense, assess and all the rest. Few youth had a vocabulary in which they could make sense of their civic engagement as political, democratic, and citizen.

All of this also matters in program assessment and evaluation, both process and outcome, around the focused goals of civic learning, citizenship education, adolescent and youth development, and community and social change. A PA example from a Kansas City, Missouri, Catholic school makes this point: "I was the one who called the Park Department. They would not talk to me. I called three times. Then I talked to my coach. We decided that I should call the City Council first and get them to help me. That worked. Later when I called the Park Department, someone spoke to me."

Is this young person talking about making a telephone call or something else? Is this telephone call a significant citizen action or just a telephone call? For this young person, this telephone call had a civic purpose and required his or her courage; it was "scary." The telephone call was made in the name of the project, to work on a public issue and was a step in addressing an important personal concern. On the surface, simply a phone call, explored more fully, is a powerful example of an everyday civic act. The observer has to be able to discern the meaning of the act to the youth; the young person must have an interpretive frame and a language to make sense out of her/his act as a civic act and of himself/herself as doing citizen.

Describing Civic Youth Work

> The practical sense of nursing is an articulation of the essence of the way in which nursing is practiced. Unfortunately, many people think of practical as methods or techniques used in practice. But methods and techniques, isolated from the systems of meaning which give direction to their use in achieving the goods at which they aim, make little sense and hence are not practical at all. (Bishop & Scudder, 1990, p. 13)

As for nursing, so too for civic youth work. Brought to civic youth work, the primary system of meaning is democratic citizenship, and the second is human development, a broader and more inclusive frame than scientific adolescent development or socially normative youth development (Rich, 1971; Rogoff, 2003). That is, the work of the civic youth worker is co-creating democratic living citizens and this, at its most robust, is a moral frame for understanding, practicing, and evaluating the human development of young people.

Analyzing a bit more, note that we wrote co-creating democratic living-citizen, not citizen as social role. Rather, the goal is to bring about living-citizen, the doing and being citizen as a mode of being-in-the-world. Yet to make this confusing, when one is citizen one can read oneself as citizen and can be so read by others. What we are getting at is that here there are two ways of making sense and these are compatible and often congruent.

This means that how the youth worker orients to the young person/people, what he or she does and how it is done must be read and make sense to them and us both as grounded, practical democratic practice and not as abstract, reified youth work. The civic youth worker craft orientation, then, is to invite a way of doing and being a self (Kotarba & Fontana, 1984), a democratic, citizen self. What the youth worker does is to try *to become present and available to actual young people as an embodied invitation to co-create here and now space/time to be together and to work together in democratic ways on some issue, problem, condition or situation of immediate interest to them*, and to do this over and over again. How this is done, the particular and specific acts, methods and procedures are quite varied and many are available (Hildreth, 1998; McIntyre, 2000), and some having been evaluated as to their effectiveness against specific outcomes (Lerner, 2004; Winter, 2003). We prefer to distinguish between what is done and how it is done. In the same way, it is how one lives that shows lived-citizen and living as citizen, not only what she or he does, such as voting. Since a citizen as such can do bad, even evil, we write democratic lived-citizen. Since that too can lead to evil or merely the bad, it becomes clear that democratic civic youth work is a moral practice and not a neutral scientific practice–a moral practice based in part on/in the sciences of adolescent development, about political life, social change, and the like.

This formulation owes much to Bishop and Scudder's (1990) work on nursing, which has a clear and single bio-medical science base for nursing science and several other sources for its philosophy, approaches, and methods. This is true too for teaching (de los Reyes & Gozemba, 2002; van Manen, 1990), social work (Healy, 2000; Nelson Reid & Popple, 1992), and other human services. In all of these, expertise is an action praxis joining values, philosophy, morality, and technique. This is why one could claim that civic youth work and related praxes are more complex practices than rocket science. Bishop and Scudder (1990) title their book on nursing, *The Practical, Moral and Personal Sense of Nursing: A Phenomenological Philosophy of Practice*. A full description of civic youth work would do the same. What remains is to give more examples along with short discussion of the practices shown.

> Yeah, well, [the worker] like, [the worker] doesn't try and be like the leader, or the head guy, [the worker] makes us like try and be that, or one of us steps in the day, and, it works out, like, usually.

> She wasn't like those [workers] that just stepped back and kind of watch us; she actually participated in this with us.

> [The worker] is like "a supervisor who's just, if you need anything like materials, whatever, they will get it for you and will not take over your project."

> Just this last time I was waving the laser in a kind of cool way and it caused, like, a weird, like, shape to appear and [the worker] was talking about it and they tried to figure out more about it. And it turns out that we couldn't really do anything cool with it. But we just, you know, [the worker] kind of like took that idea, and I felt kind of special because [the worker] was paying attention to my ideas, I guess.

For those partial to cookbooks for teaching particular skills, we suggest reviewing and adapting *Public Adventures*, by 4-H (Bass, 1999), *Building Worlds, Transforming Lives, the Public Achievement Guidebook* (Hildreth, 1998), or *Developing Communities in Partnership with Youth* (Center for Youth as Resources, 2001). Remember it is not just what is done, it is also *how* it is done and what this doing means within the context of democratic lived-citizens as a type of human development for all persons and, given our interests, young people especially.

The What and How of Civic Youth Work

The general task of civic youth work is the ongoing co-creation with young people of democratic living-citizen. How is this done? Through the ongoing embodied invitation of worker to young person. Crucial is how the worker does his/her job. How does he or she live as an open invitation to responsible working together? All of this is part of civic education and civic youth work as a type of sociopolitical pedagogy, civic education (civics). This pedagogy is more social than individual in its orientation to taking on citizen role in one's life-worlds at home, school, play and work; in its orientation to interdependency between and among others in small to large groups and in its awareness of social norms, social roles, social practices, and discourses constituting issues and ways of response. It is social in how the personal is brought to the everyday and in how freedom, choice, and responsibility–the Existential and existential triology–are given situated sociopolitical expression.

These general orientations of the craft and practice of civic education work as touchstones of reality (Friedman, 1976) that take on meaning-to-live-by in situations and other contexts. These elements of the civic youth work orientation can be made more specific.

Elements of Civic Youth Work Orientation

These elements are skill-sets or skill-clusters in the role-set (Merton, 1961) of civic youth worker. These are many ways of ordering and presenting skills basic to a semi- or full profession. This is one we prefer but may not be best for you the teacher, trainer, or worker: keep our ethos, and change the specifics!

A skill can be presented as inside or outside a situation or other context, as trained ability to master a task at a high level of competence and consistency; skill can be presented as an objective act and as a meaningful act. For us, skill is a meaningful, contextual act of expertise (Bishop & Scudder, 1990). Beyond even this, skills are embodied–we do these–and thus, along with meaning found in the craft orientation of civic youth work, skills are modes-of-doing and being lived citizen. Skills in this sense are philosophy-in-action, are praxis. Skills along with ethos and orientation are the essentials of the civic youth work craft orientation.

In presenting skills as modes of doing and being, we do not get to the level of technique, as in the chairs in the room are 17 inches apart, in a half circle, with. . . . Rather, we are at a more abstract level of skill orientation, and we use examples from interviews to point out what we want you to notice. In this we are suggesting that the workers' skills may not be visible to the naked eye. Instead, one must learn to see and hear these, to discern their presence, relevance, utility, and effectiveness. Second, we are quietly following Martin Buber's notion of teaching as pointing: "I have no teaching. I only point to something. I point to reality. I point to something in reality that had not or had too little been seen" (Schlipp & Friedman, 1967, p. 693). What are the essential modes-of-doing and being that we point to and in this way show *educaré*–opening outward, toward, i.e., educating?

Education as the "Discovery of Responsibility" (Morris, 1966)

> I mean there's a lot of things that are really difficult that probably I
> don't even know if they'll ever be able to control. But you have to try,
> and see if it does work, and if it doesn't you have to keep trying.

The worker invites young people into recognizing their responsibility to act in civic space as a way to live their freedom through choice
(Lesnoff-Caravaglia, 1972). This is part of what it means to be a citizen
in personal, social, and political terms. The worker lives a mode of doing and being either by going to the place of young people or inviting
them to another place, being clear that the purpose of coming together is
to freely explore individual and collective issues, problems, and concerns in their everyday lives or beyond in neighborhood, community,
city, nation, world. Both the explicit and implicit message is that we together will co-create safe, public space for exploration, person choice,
and group decision. In that common (civic) space, we will together
come to agreement about whether we want to continue to come together
in the hope and possibility of community–of persons, of interests, or for
other purposes.

In these ways, individual youth and the worker both live their personal and civic responsibility to choose how they want their world to be
and how they want to live so as to bring about and sustain that world.
Their choice is about co-crafting future and, in this, co-crafting self
(Holstein & Gubrium, 2000).

Education as the "Partnership of Existence" (Friedman, 1976)

> I didn't really think, like by myself, I would be able to change
> something in the community. But maybe with the group, I can. And
> so a lot of like the possibilities you can do with the group that might
> not be possible by yourself. Because then you have nobody help-
> ing you, and you're just trying to do it yourself. Now if you have
> the group, you can gather information and data, and everything,
> and have support from other people.

The worker invites young people into explicit realization that one's
moral responsibility to others is both face-to-face (Calarco, Friedman,
& Atterton, 2004) and more abstract (e.g., acting against hunger in a far
away country) and that each person can join with others in types of interdependency which makes explicit each person's responsibility to

those others, near and far. This recognizes the existential truth that "... our very existence is only properly understood as a partnership. We become selves with one another and live our lives with one another in the most real sense of the term" (Friedman, 1974, pp. 304-305). Coming together to explore common interests and purposes is a ground for recognizing that we need others and the space for living-out that recognition. Citizen is a recognition of one's place in this social and political partnership. The Civic Youth worker's invitation as a mode of doing and being civic educator embodies existential trust (Friedman, 1974) in this partnership.

Education in "Existential Trust"

> We're all connected to the same role. Like everybody had to be responsible for a different part. And then, like, if I wasn't, I would set that example and, like, seeing that I'm not responsible, not dependable.

The worker as embodied civic ethos exists as a mode of address inviting young people to respond and, by so doing, to disclose "existential trust" (Friedman, 1974) as a possibility that exists and that they can make real by choosing freely to live in this as their mode-of-being and doing. There can be no together without this, and the courage to name, decide, choose, and act in common purpose on common interest presumes each person's willingness to believe and live the promise of existential trust.

Related in the worker-young person address and response is the idea of vocation, a conversation between and acts following from a compelling world-address–person, issue, problem, situation–its being noticed and read, and one's free choice to act, to respond. The civic youth worker as educator makes explicit both existential trust and vocation as reality touchstones guiding everyday life and life in the purposive group the civic youth worker is co-forming and co-sustaining with young people.

Education as Caring

> [The workers] are pretty cool. You know, you can just have fun around [and] with them, and actually have a decent talk.

Civic youth educators live caring about and caring for (Mayerhoff, 1971; Noddings, 1984) as modes of being and doing and, in this way, point the way to individual, small group, and larger group ways of being with others. Caring here is not a thing or an attribute or a process but, instead, is a way of doing whatever one chooses to do; it is a how of doing, a quality of being together, one woven into responsibility, partnership of existence, and existential trust. Caring about individuals, issues and problems and caring for others are all included.

All civic youth work is about caring in these ways, in the invitation to come together, in how educator and young people work together and in how each makes individual and collective sense out of their togetherness: What is the meaning to each of our coming together to work together on this issue?

These four existential modes of doing and being civic youth work beg for specificity, concreteness, particularity. While we hear this, we respond in a way which is oriented to topics quietly introduced above: expertise, mastery and the skills of civic youth work. First, we introduce briefly the stage(s) of civic youth work.

From Stages of Civic Youth Work to Action-Orientation as a Stage-in-a-Process

A youth work process is constituted of smaller units, smaller time segments, and acts. Our language for this is phases or stages: earlier/later; now/then; first this, then that. Such youth work processes are not natural obviously; instead they come from practice experience and are reflected upon and later conceptualized as a process–a way of doing, the steps in doing, a praxis of purpose, way and steps, for example. Rarely, empirical research documents and evaluates such processes. Typically, processes of this type earn their legitimacy from practitioners who answer the questions, "What are you doing?" and "How do you do it?" with "This is my process"–trainers and educators too talk and write about the youth work process.

So there must be a civic youth work process!

And this is what is claimed by Banks (1999), Edgington, Kowalski, and Randall (2005), Jeffs and Smith (1999), Krueger (1980) and Maier (1987). Here words get slippery and the civic youth work process can blur into method, technique and guideline, and then come issues of expertise, mastery and skill to carry-out this process. For the moment, allow that there is a family of civic youth work processes and one way to understand these is as a sequence of stages. In this frame, we propose that there is a process composed of four sets of actions and these may occur in sequence 1-4 over a short to long period or they may occur in alternate sequences, e.g., 1,4,2,3 or 1,3,2,4. The actual sequence is decided upon by the worker and the young people in each specific context.

Action Sets:

1. Entering the place (site).
2. Co-creating the place (site) as a democratic civic rehearsal space.
3. Co-sustaining the democratic space at that place (site).
4. Co-expanding the democratic space into the larger world.

The civic youth worker must do 1 and, if she has been working with these same young people for some time, she may also and, at the same time, work at 3. Put academically, a distinction between when an act in a process sequence is undertaken can be distinguished from the intention of the act, and these may be incongruent. There can be simultaneity in the acts as seen from afar while, internally and phenomenologically, the intention of 1 and 3 are clearly different.

All of this is also about strategies, tactics, expertise, mastery, and skills–all in the context of what is civic youth work, what is its purpose, what are its approach and methods, and how do its practitioners go about their work (purpose, activities, acts and the rest). Let's examine this next using a constructed example based in our direct practice and research.

There is essentially only one stage of practice in civic youth work–the beginning. The beginning is entered or brought about over and over, always with the same purpose–to again co-create communal, civic space for work together on issues, problems and concerns important and meaningful to the young people participating. This is not non-sense! Instead, it is our effort to move toward *ever renewed beginning* as the way of this work and, in so doing, move away from a cookbook approach or a handbook or method that guides the worker through a process presumed to be, but rarely proven, effective: first stage is introduction, the second problem-finding and so on.

However, there is something important about such guides, training manuals, handbooks and cookbooks; they indeed can guide. But they alone are not the work of civic youth work–*the how of the way one does together*. This is the work, the praxis; and the work is done always as depending, as contingent on who is there, previously together-work, real-world constraints and openings, and the rest.

What Does the Civic Youth Worker Have to Know About and Have to Be Able to Do?

The civic youth worker walks into a room where six teenagers are sitting, talking, listening on their headphones. It is in a middle school and the young people are students in the school. They came to the room to join a group called Students for a Better School. Six hundred students could have come at this time to participate in this group; they receive no school credit for being involved; their effort will be recorded on their school record and on their report card, which their parents must sign and return to the school.

1. What does the civic youth worker see?

- Kids, teens, young people, adolescents?
- 12, 13, 14 year olds?
- Good/bad kids?
- Caucasian, African American, Hispanic, Asian-American, African kids?
- Tall/short, skinny/fat, just right bodies?
- Volunteers, potential participants?
- Citizens?

Civic youth work-in-practice begins before the worker comes to the door; the worker knows as much as possible about: the purpose of the meeting; who called it and why; that person's role in the school; why she or he and not someone else called the meeting; the history of such efforts in general, in schools, with young people this age, in this community and city, etc. She has done some homework and can place this in more inclusive, more complex, and more useful contexts: she knows a lot about this sort of event, space and participants. She comes informed.

What does she do with all of this information, this preparation?

She puts it all into parenthesis (van Manen, 1990) and goes into the room and towards the young people as if one has never before done this. Why?

So that the uniqueness of this situation with these specific young people will have a chance to show the worker what and who they are in their particularity and uniqueness. She wants to be able to work here for the first time–the moment when everything is new and fresh and full of possibility.

Does one forget what is known?

No, merely sets these aside, for now.

2. What does one do next?

She says "hi" and introduces herself, then asks them all why they are there. She confirms the general purpose of getting together and then meets each young person. Then and there, as fully as possible (Friedman, 1983). Together they talk about why this group is being formed. And so on.

3. What is the worker orienting to and attending to?

The civic youth worker is orienting to what could emerge right now, here, with these young people regarding their coming together as a group, their working together on an issues meaningful and important to them, etc. In effect, it is orienting to future-making out of the immediate present here and now, attending to:

- The words and meanings of each person
- The body of each person
- The tone of the group, its ambience
- The sequence of the talk–who is talking, saying what, how and who speaks next, saying what, how.

The worker is imagining the possibilities of co-creating and inhabiting new spaces in which she and they make a new present, and new futures.

4. What is the worker listening for?

She is listening for opportunities to invite them to become a group, invite them to choose to work on a common issue, etc.

What does this mean? How do you listen for opportunities?

It means that the worker subjects every word, silence and body movement, every moment, to a question: Do I now invite them to work together? Do I now invite them to reflect on their talk? Do I now...? Remember: All civic youth work is co-creating beginnings!

5. What does one do next?

The civic youth worker invites and invites again and again, and again: she invites six young people to do something together, here and now such as forming a group or picking an issue to work on.

6. When does one use what has been put in the parenthesis?

The civic youth worker moves in and out of setting aside what is known from education, training, work/life experience, and the bringing it forward and using it. The more one defines herself as a professional and practices within those terms, the more reflexive you are. She is also reflective, waiting a bit, perhaps a moment or longer at the end of the meeting, to review what was done, what else could have been done and, of course, what was missed, done well and poorly. Civic youth workers evaluate to improve their practice.

As a professional she is accountable and responsible to self and others–teachers, parents, community–for the work. Thus the worker practices reflexively and reflectively (Schon, 1983) because it is an ethical imperative for professionals, because it is a good, because she may be required to do so by her agency, and because this is one way to monitor and improve practice. A good worker will also do this with young people for herself, her practice, and for theirs.

In the actual moment with the six young people, the worker watches herself watch, listens to herself think and talk, always aware of one's own awareness and of whatever is going on. During these moments of awareness, the worker can bring forward learning–education, training, experience–to make sense out of what is going on with two purposes: (1) the co-creating and co-sustaining with these young people here and now of civic space; and (2) the healthy development of these young people.

What grounds our example is the context, the situation, the stage in the process, the worker's stance (ethos), craft orientation, and praxis. A traditional language for these is knowledge, attitudes, and skills. We want to explore next how the categories of knowledge, skills, and attitudes can be reframed and to suggest positive consequences of this for civic youth work practice and for understanding it.

EXPERTISE, MASTERY, TECHNIQUE, AND SKILLS: WHAT IS CIVIC YOUTH WORK?

The classical frame for doing, understanding and researching practice in the applied human, social, and behavioral sciences–education, social work, counseling, and the like is to show relevant practitioner knowledge, attitudes, and skills. At times, these latter are grounded in methods and techniques. This is the frame of applied science contrasted by Bishop and Scudder (1990) to "practical human science." Without walking this distinction back to epistemology, tradition, and culture in the crafts, arts and sciences–where there are real, important and complex issues–we nudge up against these complexities by examining civic youth work as expertise, mastery, and skills. We embed skills, as Bishop and Scudder, Jr. (1990) suggest, in meanings. Simply put, skill is practiced, animated, brought into existence in its performance, and that is always in a place, at a time, in a situation and in other contexts–skill is a situated act.

A skill is a particular type of act; its home is in two language and related social worlds–the workplace and mastery and expertise. The home of a skill is disclosed in answer to the question, "What does it take to do this job?" (Simon, Schenke, & Dippo, 1991, p. 27). A skill is not the sole possession of an individual or even individuals in a "community of practice" or a field or profession. Rather, skills are "always dependent for their development, display and maintenance on opportunities to put them into practice" (Simon, Schenke, & Dippo, 1991, p. 45). To get at skills, first get at the situation and the work-at-hand: What is the work/job to be done? What does it take to get the job done?

This is where skill is to be found. To look other places is to risk reifying skill, that is, treating it, an abstraction, as a concrete, particular thing or activity. A second home for skill is qualitative, not defining. It is about skill performance. Both skill and mastery are inside the larger frame of expertise (Ericsson & Smith, 1991). In the context of civic youth work skill, technique, mastery, and expertise are performative-in-context of what is at-hand to be done. Skills join in its performance, as well as do ethos, stance, orientation.

Beyond all of this, skill is a mode of doing/being. This means that skill is not only realized in performance as praxis; skill is also a way of living–the joining of one's doing and being. This is true especially in our society where what we do is said to be who we are, that is, doing drives being.

Further, skill is one element of technique and both are essential to "practical science" (Strasser, 1985). In practical science seen phenomenologically, the intentionality of the worker brings together what is needed to do a job (p. 57); the civic youth worker is a practical person and brings together what is needed to do this job here and now–with these youth in this venue with one and a half hours to get it done. This practical person brings together knowledge of young people as such; democratic, civic values and practices; the setting; the stage of the process and the like so as to craft in the here and now intentional acts to co-create, co-sustain, and co-extend young people's civic engagement.

Education and Training

Since skill in these senses is a verb, is action (in the service of a task), a performance, then mastery and expertise are high levels of performance. This tells us that the education and training of civic youth work skills is best done in an experiential pedagogy–learning quality performance through practice (Argyris, 1993; Argyris & Schon, 1974). But of a particular kind: each civic youth work skill then is a cluster of meanings, acts, activities, knowing, beliefs specific to each unique context and situation in which there is work to be done. What is the work to be done? Learning to do and be living-citizens in specially constructed rehearsal spaces and also in the larger worlds of school, neighborhood, community and beyond.

What is in this cluster? Again: belief in inclusive and just living-citizenship, understanding young person as human being and life moment-in-context, how to rightly and correctly work to co-create and co-sustain a democratic civic space, and the like.

How should civic youth workers be prepared? Doing with them exactly what one wants them to do with young people and doing this with an unusually high degree of explicitness about intention, purpose, technique, and evaluation so that the worker can come to understand as both insider (group member) and outsider (teacher) the reasoning for each element of the work. Doing this will facilitate the worker's own evaluation of the work, of self, of youth, and the ongoing enhancement of the work. This also is true in all accounts for the worker doing action-research (McNiff & Whitehead, 2006; Stringer, 1996) in addition to–or rather than–process and/or outcome evaluation.

CONCLUSION

Civic youth work is proposed as a new craft orientation for preparing young people for living-citizenship and for working on issues and policies supporting their everyday involvement in school, community, job site, and spiritual place. Introduced and outlined were the craft orientation and ethos, major skills/modes of being and doing, and the civic youth work process.

We conclude with a call for serious analysis, reflection, and action on civic youth work as such and on the need for it because of the moral panic about youth as citizens, because of the political right young people have to participate in issues that concern and affect them, because young people say these opportunities are valuable and meaningful, because of the relative failure of traditional civics education, because of the relative success of the experiential education pedagogy, and because few in mainline child and youth care, education, or related professions are doing the daily, never-ending work of preparing young people to be just, nonviolent, and responsible agents in and for civil society now as youth and later as adults.

Somebody has to do this public work with and in the name of and for democracy! As Hanna Arendt, the political philosopher wrote, "The primary source of meaning and action . . . [is] in democratic action" (Ingram, 2006, p. 37).

REFERENCES

Argyris, C. (1993). Knowledge for action: A guide to overcoming barriers to organizational change. San Francisco: Jossey-Bass Inc.

Argyris, C., & Schon, D. (1974). Theory in practice: Increasing professional effectiveness. San Francisco: Jossey-Bass.

Banks, J. (1997). Educating citizens in a multicultural society. New York: Teachers College Press.

Bass, M. (1999). Public adventures guides handbook: An active citizenship curriculum for youth. Minneapolis, MN: 4-H Cooperative Curriculum System.

Bishop, A. H., & Scudder, J. R. (1990). Practical, moral, and personal sense of nursing: A phenomenological philosophy of practice. Albany, NY: State University of New York Press.

Boyte, H., & Skelton, N. (1997). The legacy of public work: Education for citizenship. Educational Leadership, 54(5), 12-18.

Butts, R. F. (1980). The revival of civic learning: A rationale for citizenship education in.

Calarco, M., Friedman, M., & Atterton, P. (Eds.). (2004). Levinas and Buber: Dialogue and difference. Pittsburg: Duquesne University Press.

Carse, J. (1986). Finite and infinite games. New York: Free Press. American schools. Bloomington, IN: Phi Delta Kappa Educational Foundation.

Center for Youth as Resources. (2001). Developing communities in partnership with youth: A manual for starting and maintaining youth as resources programs. Washington, DC: Center for Youth as Resources.

de los Reyes, E., & Gozemba, P. (2002). Pockets of hope: How students and teachers change the world. Westport, CT: Bergin & Garvey.

Dewey, J. (1938). Experience and education. New York: Collier Books.

Edginton, C., Kowalski, C., & Randall, S. (2005). Youth Work: Emerging perspectives in youth development. Champaign, IL: Sagamore Publishing, L.L.C.

Ericsson, K., & Smith, J. (Eds.). (1991). Toward a general theory of expertise: prospects and limits. Cambridge: Cambridge University Press.

Friedman, M. (1974). Touchstones of reality: Existential trust and the community of peace. New York: E.P. Dutton & Co., Inc.

Friedman, M. (1976). Martin Buber: The life of dialogue. Chicago: University of Chicago Press.

Friedman, M. (1983). The confirmation of otherness in family, community and society. New York: The Pilgrim Press.

Healy, K. (2000). Social work practices: Contemporary perspectives on change. Thousand Oaks, CA: Sage Publications.

Hildreth, R. (1998). Building worlds, transforming lives, making history: A guide to public achievement. Minneapolis, MN: The Center for Democracy and Citizenship.

Holstein, J., & Gubrium, J. (2000). The self we live by: Narrative identity in a postmodern world. New York: Oxford University Press.

Ingram, D. (2006). Hanna Arendt. In J. Protevi (Ed.), *A dictionary of continental philosophy*. New Haven, CT: Yale University Press.

Jeffs, T. (2001). Citizenship, youth work and democratic renewal. Scottish Youth Issues Journal, 2(1), 11-34.

Jeffs, T., & Smith, M. (1999). Informal education: Conversation, democracy and learning. Derbyshire, UK: Education Now Publishing Co-operative Limited.

Joplin, L. (1995). On defining experiential education. In K. Warren, M. Sakofs, & J. Hunt, Jr. (Eds.). The theory of experiential education. Dubuque, IA: Kendall/Hunt Publishing Company.

Kolb, D. (1984). Experiential learning: Experience as the source of learning and development. Englewood Cliffs, NJ: Prentice-Hall, Inc.

Kotarba, J., & Fontana, A. (1984). The existential self in society. Chicago: The University of Chicago Press.

Krueger, M. (1980). Intervention techniques for child care workers. Milwaukee, WI: James F. Tall, Publisher.

Lerner, R. (2004). Liberty: Thriving and civic engagement among America's youth. Thousand Oaks, CA: Sage Publications.

Lesnoff-Caravaglia, G. (1972). Education as existential possibility. New York: Philosophical Library.

Maier, H. W. (1987). Developmental group care of children and youth: Concepts and practice. New York: The Haworth Press.

Mayeroff, M. (1971). On caring. New York: HarperCollins Publishers.

McIntyre, A. (2000). Inner-city kids: Adolescents confront life and violence in an urban community. New York: New York University Press.

McNiff, J., & Whitehead, J. (2006). All you need to know about action research. Thousand Oaks, CA: Sage Publications, Inc.

Morris, V. C. (1966). Existentialism in education. New York: Harper & Row.

Nelson Reid, P., & Popple, P. (1992). The moral purpose of social work: The character and intensions of a profession. Chicago: Nelson-Hall Publishers.

Noddings, N. (1984). Caring: A feminine approach to ethics and moral education. Berkeley and Los Angeleos: University of California Press.

Patrick, J. (1996). Principles of Democracy for the Education of Citizens. In J. Patrick & L. Pinhey (Eds.), Resources on civic education for democracy: International perspectives (pp. 5-17). Bloomington, ID: ERIC Clearinghouse for International Civic Education.

Rich, J. (1971). Humanistic foundations of education. Worthington, OH: Charles A. Jones Publishing Company.

Rogoff, B. (2003). The cultural nature of human development. New York: Oxford University Press.

Schon, D. (1983). The reflective practitioner: How professionals think in action. New York: Basic Books.

Schlipp, P., & Friedman, M. (1967). The philosophy of Martin Buber. Lasalle, IL: Open Court.

Simon, R., Schenke, A., & Dippo, D. (1991). Learning work: A critical pedagogy of work education. New York: Bergin and Garvey.

Strasser, S. (1985). Understanding and explanation: Basic ideas concerning the humanity of the human sciences. Pittsburgh, PA: Duquesne University Press.

Stringer, E. (1996). Action research: A handbook for practitioners. Thousand Oaks, CA: Sage Publications, Inc.

van Manen, M. (1990). Researching lived experience: Human science for an action sensitive pedagogy. Ontario, Canada: The Althouse Press.

Winter, N. (2003, April 24). Social capital, civic engagement and positive youth development outcomes. Retrieved January 2, 2006, from http://www.policystudies.com/studies/community/Civic%20Engagement.pdf

Index

For Product Safety Concerns and Information please contact our EU
representative GPSR@taylorandfrancis.com
Taylor & Francis Verlag GmbH, Kaufingerstraße 24, 80331 München, Germany